Other Books by the Author

Pediatrics: Some Uncommon Views on Some Common Problems

Sandy, We Love You

Professionally Speaking: Public Speaking for Health Professionals

Medical Writing 101: A Primer for Health Professionals

Parenthood: Laugh and Understand Your Child

Ethical Problems in Pediatrics: A Dozen Dilemmas

Arnold Melnick, DO, MSc, DHL (Hon.), FACOP

Bloomington, IN  Milton Keynes, UK

authorHOUSE®

AuthorHouse™
1663 Liberty Drive, Suite 200
Bloomington, IN 47403
www.authorhouse.com
Phone: 1-800-839-8640

AuthorHouse™ UK Ltd.
500 Avebury Boulevard
Central Milton Keynes, MK9 2BE
www.authorhouse.co.uk
Phone: 08001974150

First published by AuthorHouse 2/14/2007

ISBN: 978-1-4259-9206-4 (sc)

Library of Congress Control Number: 2007900629

Printed in the United States of America
Bloomington, Indiana

This book is printed on acid-free paper.

Dedication

To my parents, to my school teachers, to my
medical school trainers and to my colleagues,
who by precept, mentoring and example,
inculcated in me a sense of ethics that has
lasted a lifetime. To them all, I say,
"Thank You!".

Table of Contents

Introduction

Mention the word "ethics" to most people and it conjures up a panoply of situations, all commonly associated with such problems as issues of death, withholding of therapy, abortion, beginning of life and right to die, among others.

Active health professionals, whether captains of the ship – such as physicians or dentists—or other professionals, such as optometrists, podiatrists, psychologists, pharmacists – or other members of the health team, such as nurses, technicians, aides and the like—sooner or later, to a greater or lesser extent, will find themselves personally involved in some ethical problem or moral or value judgment.

But there are situations in children and adolescents which are not as intense or gut-wrenching but perhaps equally important. Either the captain of the care team or other health professionals might be the involved professional. That professional may be the first one involved, or the one the child has enough confidence in to make the initial approach. But the response must be grounded in good value judgments.

That's what this book is all about.

I have compiled a series of situations (some actual, some manufactured to illustrate a point) in which a child may be involved -- relatively common situations. On the page following each one, I have presented a set of possible actions for the reader to choose from. That is deliberate. You, the reader, can read each problem and, without the influence of "answers" on the same page, consider what you think are the possible – or best -- solutions for all concerned. Then you can select from the list presented. Following this, I have added my comments for each solution, and then a general analysis of the situation, titled Ethical Considerations. These value-judgment situations create a form of self-teaching that, even in print, is also in an interactive mode.

If you want to stretch your mind even farther, figure out what you believe is the need, rationale, impact and effect of every solution offered—not just the one you select as best. This will allow you to ruminate over a number of ethical choices and broaden your viewpoint on value judgments.

Solutions are not necessarily "right" or "wrong," so we won't always agree.

At the same time, remember that many solutions are based on ethical principles (such as patient confidentiality, first do not harm, patient autonomy) or moral principles (such as truthfulness, not destroying hope, application of the Golden Rule) or both. And all involve professional value judgments.

In every situation, try to be sure that your solution causes the least pain, solves the problem to the greatest extent, upholds your responsibility as a health professional, and does not encroach upon societal restrictions. And most important for me is the one that provides the greatest help and solace to the child involved. In other words, you must think about each situation!

So, read, think, and have fun.

Second Opinions

At the end of each chapter, following my discussions of the ethics involved in each case, you will find a commentary that I hope will add to your knowledge and your thinking. It will present another view of the ethics of the situation and may agree or not agree with my opinion of the ethics

I am deeply indebted to these colleagues for their second opinions:

Cyril Blavo, DO, MS, MPH & TM, FACOP – Professor of Pediatrics and Public Health, and Director of the Public Health Program, College of Osteopathic Medicine, Nova Southeastern University.

Stanley Cohen, EdD - Vice Provost, Health Professions Division; Professor and Chairman, Division of Medical Humanities, College of Osteopathic Medicine; both at Nova Southeastern University.

Edward A. Packer, DO, FAAP, FACOP – Chairman, Department of Pediatrics, College of Osteopathic Medicine, Nova Southeastern University, and Program Director, Pediatric Residency Program, Palms West Hospital.

Kenneth E. Johnson, DO, FACOOG – Associate Professor, Department of Obstetrics/Gynecology and Public Health, and Director, Women's Health Clinic, College of Osteopathic Medicine, Nova Southeastern University.

Frank DePiano, PhD – Vice President for Academic Affairs and Founding Dean, Center for Psychological Studies, both at Nova Southeastern University.

Robert Locke, DO, FACOP – Division of Neonatology, Clinical Associate Professor of Pediatrics, Christiana Hospital/A.I. DuPont Hospital for Children, Thomas Jefferson University School of Medicine.

Stanley E. Grogg, DO, FACOP – Professor of Pediatrics, Oklahoma State University – Center for Health Sciences.

Samuel K. Snyder, DO, FACOI, FACP, FASN – Chairman, Department of Internal Medicine, and Director, Division of Nephrology, College of Osteopathic Medicine, Nova Southeastern University

Sandy D. Melnick, MD – Attending Psychiatrist and Director of Outpatient Psychotherapy, Chester-Crozer Medical Center.

In each instance, I chose a professional colleague who had a wide perspective of ethics and a knowledge base related to the specific subject. Each one had training and experience to produce a learned and objective second opinion. None were told what to say, so that their commentaries are totally theirs, subject only to technical editing.

These contributors exceeded what was expected of them. They all added breadth to the ethical interpretations as well as depth of insight, plus substantial thought and valuable ideas. For all this, I am grateful.

Situation One

John is a 14-year old you have taken care of almost since birth. You have a splendid relationship with him and with his family. He comes to your office one day without his parents and asks to speak with you in total confidence.

He says he believes he has gonorrhea (later confirmed). You know that, if his parents find out, there will be a tremendous family upheaval. What do you do?

The Options

1. Call his parents and tell them.

2. Try to convince him to notify his parents and to accept the consequences.

3. Treat him in confidence and bill his parents.

4. Treat him in confidence and make no charge.

5. Refer him to a clinic.

A Look at the Options

1. Call his parents and tell them

When John came in, he asked to speak in strict confidence. Since he did speak to you, we must assume you agreed to this confidence. Therefore, it is a gross violation of professional trust to "go behind his back" and notify his parents. About the only mitigating factor in violating a trust would be the threat of death, suicide or murder. Then, the health professional is obligated to report it.

Even if calling his parents were not so egregious an act, that patient would be lost to you forever. He would never again trust you or anything you say—and that might even interfere with some future diagnostic plan or therapeutic suggestion. Or even keep him from coming to you at all when he has another illness. And you may be sure that once he reaches his maturity—or even before if he can influence his parents—he will leave you behind as his physician. Loss of a patient from your practice should never influence your decisions. That's materialistic. That's financial. And those factors should not dictate how you act, professionally or ethically. So, you don't choose options based on that.

In some instances, a physician may say to himself, "I would like to help this young man, but if I don't tell his parents and they find out, they will all leave my practice—and that's several patients I'll lose." This is purely self-serving and should never enter the equation. The ethical—and the professional—question must be: All things considered, what is the best solution in the long run for all concerned?

In other situations, the physician might take an autocratic view. I know best. Or only the child's parents know best. Or why should I help him out and possibly get myself into trouble? Or even worse: He got himself into that situation, why is it my concern? Why should I try to get him out of it? Let him take his punishment.

But it is not unusual for health professionals to help a patient even when it means slight bending of the truth or double-talking to a third party. We must remember that the person we are treating is the patient, not the parent, not the spouse, not the employer. We owe our full professional care to the patient, regardless of who engages us or who pays the bills. Often, this is a difficult concept for practicing professionals. Look at it this way:

Assume that it is John's father who contracts gonorrhea, and he is covered by Union Eclectic Insurance Company. You treat him, and his insurance company demands more than the minimum information, information that really is privileged, that is confidential between patient and doctor. Rare indeed is the physician who would violate the confidence of the patient just because the entity paying the bill demands it. Similarly, the child is the patient, not the parent, and he's the one for whom the doctor is responsible.

Over and above the ethical matters, in the state of Florida and perhaps in other states, it is illegal to notify the parents in such instances (Figure 1).

2. Try to convince him to notify his parents and to accept the consequences

In almost all instances, the best solution for a problem is openness and honesty. The fewer secrets and the less hidden information, the more comfortable everyone will be in the long run. Probably this is even more true when between parents and children. The impact is there when a parent keeps a secret from a child (and most of them do) but explosive when a child keeps from a parent information as important as John's bout with gonorrhea. On that basis, this seems to be the appropriate solution.

However, you start with the knowledge that when they find out, there will be a tremendous upheaval. Invectives. Accusations. Recriminations. All the negatives. Two things have to be done.

First, John must be prepared to accept the parental reactions and punishments. Many times, the imagined reaction will not be as bad, when all is said and done, as one might expect. Sometimes it is worse. If you, the health practitioner, have any ethical or moral feeling of responsibility, you will (in addition to your medical treatment) spend a few sessions (whatever is necessary) with John. Explain the possible reaction from his parents. Emotionally support him. Let him know that you are willing to sit down with John and his parents. If he persistently refuses, you have no choice but to go to another plan.

When you get John and his parents together, you can be a buffer, if you act fairly: explain the situation to the parents, review the alternatives, and discuss the possible punishments. Throughout, keep the sessions under control and well modulated. Encourage all of them to discuss the situation as calmly as possible and help them to reach an equitable solution. Offer to refer them (not just John) to an appropriate mental health counselor (psychiatrist, psychologist, social worker) if severe tension persists and if you do not feel qualified to handle this type of problem.

Your action will lead to adequate and open medical treatment of the gonorrhea, to reestablishment of the family unit with trust, and, for all of them, to more acceptance and comfort with the situation. You have saved a young man, acted in a way that will set a fine example (of handling problems) for his future life, and salvaged a terrible situation by saving a family.

Do not let money or consideration of money get in the way of your actions..

3. *Treat him in confidence and bill his parents*

All that was said about confidentiality in the first option applies here. Confidence is obviously violated if you send the parents a bill. Review the discussion from Option 1 and read carefully the applicable sections from Florida law (Figure 1). Other states may have similar regulations.

The billing becomes another matter. Students and physicians discussing this option often ask the question, "Who is going to pay for the treatment?" That's important because payment for services is how a health professional makes his or her income. However, the crux of the problem should not be money; it should be concern for a patient who needs treatment. Your patient. Your patient for many years. Your patient who probably would not know where to turn if you reject him.

Some have suggested that if you decide not to tell his parents, a payment schedule for the treatment should be worked out directly with John, either cash payments (from some sort of odd jobs) or having him do odd jobs for the doctor. "This will be so that he learns the lesson that he must pay for his mistakes. That will teach him for the future." I believe that it is not the function of the health professional "to teach John a lesson" or "to make him pay for his mistakes." Option 2 will take care of that.

But if you feel that money is a consideration, think of this: You have treated him for years. You have collected fees from his parents for years. Would it upset anyone's finances for you to treat him for this episode for free and save a child in the process—and maybe a family --your patients --whose allegiance to you will probably be greatly increased because of this.

4. Treat him in confidence and make no charge

Absent the opportunity to get the family together, to discuss the total situation openly and frankly and to try to restore the family unity, this seems to be the best choice.

In this option, you have preserved John's confidence by not notifying his parents. You have extended this by not billing. Billing would be a violation of that confidence. John will get his treatment, and except for the secrecy involved, this option seems to solve all aspects of the dilemma.

I believe that in this instance, your ethical obligation is to counsel John, explain the difficulties which could arise, the problems he may face and the implications of the entire situation. He needs to express his understandings and his feelings and his worries. He may need your help with these. And here is more time of yours without payment for services.

Go back to Option 3 for a more thorough discussion of the question of payment.

What we have left is two things: One, John will have to carry this secret with him forever or at least until he's an adult. Two, you (and maybe some office personnel) will have to carry the secret also. Where's the rub? Secrets have a way of slipping out sometimes. A chance remark. A forgetful moment. A wrong answer. An innuendo. There is no absolute way to guarantee that the secret will be kept. And if it is exposed at some time, much of the family dynamics can (or will) be disrupted. Distrust for John? Distrust for you? Hatred for John? Hatred for you? Who knows?

5. Refer him to a clinic

This is a form of rejection and can send shuddering thoughts through John. "This is so terrible even my favorite doctor doesn't want to have anything to do with me." "I must really be bad, he's sending me away." "What will they do to me in that clinic?" "Will the clinic call my parents?"

Option 2 can be the answer if John will cooperate. Option 4 will be a good reserve if he doesn't. Therefore, there seems to be no reason for this option—sending him away. If the parents find out, what reason will you give for rejecting their son---your patient for so long?

If there is some real reason you cannot handle this situation or don't want to (more than just "I don't want to be bothered"), a referral might be considered to a suitable clinic or a sensitive colleague—with a complete explanation to them. You owe John that much.

Figure 1
[from statutes of the State of Florida]
384.30 Minors' consent to treatment. --

(1) The department or its authorized representatives, each physician licensed to practice medicine under the provisions of chapter 458 or chapter 459, each health care professional licensed under the provisions of chapter 464 who is acting pursuant to the scope of his license, and each public or private hospital, clinic, or other health facility may examine and provide treatment for sexually transmissible diseases to any minor, if the physician, health care professional, or facility is qualified to provide such treatment. The consent of the parents or guardians of a minor is not a prerequisite for an examination or treatment.

(2) The fact of consultation, examination, and treatment of a minor for a sexually transmissible disease is confidential and shall not be divulged in any direct or indirect manner, such as sending a bill for services rendered to a parent or guardian, except as provided in s.384.29. Such information is exempt from ss.119.01 and 119.07. This exemption is subject to the Open Government Sunset Review Act in accordance with s 119.14.

Ethical Considerations

This particular case has several important aspects. It is a single incident (the gonorrhea). The medical problem can, in most instances, be cleared up readily and simply. It can be taken care of without involvement of too many people. And the child's life can be put back on track.

On the other hand, not getting the necessary therapy could ruin the child's life medically. If the physician refuses to give treatment, add rejection by a trusted adult to the child's already heavy burden. Violating the child's confidence is another form of rejection, leading to loss of trust. Teenagers, mostly because of their generally good health and their frequent feeling of omnipotence, are known to make very few doctor visits during adolescence. If rejected by a trusted physician, there is little likelihood that adolescents will seek out another doctor, a stranger, an unknown. The disease may not get treated until it is beyond simple therapy.

The doctor's (or the other health professional's) obligation —morally, ethically and professionally—is to treat the problem, maintain the necessary confidences and salvage the child. Here is a good analogy: A child on a swing is showing off, doing dangerous tricks. She falls and fractures her arm. No doctor would refuse to treat because "she brought it on herself." It is not our responsibility, as health professionals, to decide whether the child should be punished, or what punishment should be meted out, or even initiate it by reporting to the parents. And if a doctor lets his fees direct his actions, he is lacking responsibility and inflicting punishment.

One complicating factor has not been discussed. It opens too many doors and will confuse the major issue. That factor considers what to do with others who have a stake in the issue: the girl from whom he contracted the gonorrhea; siblings; other sexual contacts;, and the public health department. For the sake of this presentation, we have neutralized them. Perhaps the reader might like to set up a totally new ethical hypothesis, a new situation and new options.

Our responsibility to the parents is to do the best possible things for the patient, in our medical judgment. And that is our responsibility to the patient also. There have been legal precedents for suing doctors when, in their best judgment, a child requires surgery and the parents refuse. Courts have said that doctors must insist in the face of a medical necessity. In some states, such as Florida, refusal by the parents is considered child neglect.

The best scenario brings all parties—health professional, parents and patient—together, if possible, and without any dire consequences to any of them. We must treat as needed, support as indicated, and try to get the child a maturing experience from the situation.

Second Opinion

by Cyril Blavo, DO, MS, MPH &TM, FACOP
Professor of Pediatrics and Public Health
Director of Public Health Program
College of Osteopathic Medicine
Nova Southeastern University

Ethical issues, by their very nature, often result in a dilemma; that is, what may be perceived as right and wrong may exist to a certain extent on both sides of the issue. The challenges one faces usually call upon one's social mores, ethical principles, and moral values at times, as well as legal and professional constraints. Decisions made in the face of an ethical dilemma usually have consequences, which may be favorable to one party yet unfavorable to another.

The real challenge, therefore, is to make that decision or take that action which will maximize your resolve, that is, which will fulfill the needs of the individual to whom you are giving assistance and maintain your professional standards, without significantly compromising your moral values and ethical principles. You must, however, demonstrate some respect for the party to whom your decision may present some degree of adversity. Above all, you must abide by the law.

In that context, I would make the following determinations on this case:

- John is ill. He has acquired an infection, which needs treatment. Treatment is clearly needed and, in my view, not a part of the dilemma.
- John has some fear of reprisal from his parents (whether perceived or real) for his actions. He has engaged in sexual activity, which has resulted in his acquiring a sexually transmitted disease.
- John prefers to keep this information from his parents. The reason for his decision must be sought out.
- Does the treatment under consideration (i.e., intramuscular Ceftriaxone) carry a level of risk which warrants prior parental consent?
- What is the likely impact of treating John confidentially, at the risk of his parents discovering your action at a later date? In this case, should they find out later, there might be a loss in parental confidence in the clinician, and possible withdrawal of John as a patient.
- What is the likely impact of breaching John's confidentiality and informing his parents? In this case, possible loss of John as a patient, or discouragement of John to seek medical treatment in the future for want of trust of clinicians.
- What is the best approach to this particular problem, knowing this family, and being aware of their culture and family dynamics? How severe would the reprisal be if John changed his mind and agreed to the clinician's intervention, as an

advocate, with his parents, prior to administering the treatment?

- Are there protections under the law for administering treatment for a sexually transmitted disease to a minor without parental consent?

The reality is that John has already engaged in sexual activity and has acquired an infection. He must be treated. He has approached the health care provider for care. This must be honored. He has requested confidentiality on the matter of his diagnosis and treatment. It should be seriously considered. By addressing John's concerns the clinician is already informed about his activity, and by confirming his diagnosis the clinician is already informed about his condition.

Irrespective of the probable protection under the law for treatment of a minor without parental consent, John needs to be advised and counseled (not lectured to) about the clinician's preference. My preference would be to be an advocate for John by counseling him about his high-risk behavior and its adverse consequences. I would advocate for him by telling his parents about adolescence, and assure them that I would arrange for counseling in hope of preventing such behavior from recurring. If John is still insistent on confidentiality, I would explore his reasons so that I can appreciate any adverse situation at home which I may not be aware of, but which I may be able to intervene on in a different context. I would, nevertheless, treat John and honor the confidentiality, document my efforts at negotiating communication with his parents, and take some time to talk to him seriously about his high-risk behavior. I would also advise him to seek counseling at school (which is often confidential).

The possible consequences of treating John without the consent of his parents are

- If the treatment results in injury to John, the clinician may face liability for lack of consent (unless protected by law).
- If his parents later discover the clinician's actions, they may lose confidence in his care and no longer use his services.
- If his parents later discover that John had opted not to inform them, it may hurt their relationship with him. The fact that John went to the clinician without informing his parents is itself a potential problem.

Beyond treating John medically, I would pay greater attention to John's social and psychological well-being, offer support and education to his family and hope that John is assured of their support, even under adverse circumstances. My two major roles in this endeavor are first to be his caregiver, and then to be his advocate.

Situation Two

Lucille is a 16-year old patient whom you have seen for several years. She is intelligent, and street smart. She tells you she is sexually active and would like for you to prescribe contraceptives. What do you do?

The Options

1. Call her parents.

2. Refer her to Planned Parenthood.

3. Tell her how disappointed you are in her.

4. Prescribe contraceptives and bill her family.

5. Prescribe contraceptives and charge her.

6. Prescribe contraceptives and forget about the bill.

A Look at the Options

1. Call her parents

While Lucille did not ask for confidentiality, either in advance or at the time of the visit, you could assume that you have no obligation about notifying her parents. But the issue of confidentiality still exists. Since the situation indicates that you have cared for her for several years, I would assume that you know something about the child-parent relationships, the social status of the family, their finances and the history of any siblings. You should thus have a pretty good idea of the family's attitudes toward sexual activity, contraceptives and unwanted pregnancies.

Your actions should be based on that knowledge. Some families would be devastated and torn asunder in this situation. Others might tend to be more liberal in views, either philosophically or because of previous incidents. Some might be indifferent. The reality of the situation should be your concern for what is best for this young girl.

Breaking confidentiality and calling her parents would not stop her sexual activity, but would destroy her confidence in you. She would probably never return to you and, because she is an adolescent, most likely not go to another health professional. It certainly would fracture her relationship with her parents. Or the worst effect: she rebels, forgets about contraception and ultimately becomes pregnant.

But the initial interview, either way, calls for careful discussion of the possibilities in a calm, friendly, non-judgmental and unhurried manner. Never forget, however, the potential medical problems and see that this young girl is checked for them -- and protected against them.

If she accepts your suggestion for conferencing and counseling, the prescription of contraceptives can wait until then. If not, you must take another tack.

2. Refer her to Planned Parenthood

This could be seen as a form of rejection. However, if you fully explain that this is not your type of work, or that you feel uncomfortable in this field, or that others are better able to help--and you indicate that you are doing this because you are interested in her and supportive of her, this could be a successful referral. But beware of curt, brief and cold (or even hostile) referrals. Since she is your patient, you might convince her of your continuing interest by asking her to call and let you know how she is doing with them.

3. Tell her how disappointed you are in her.

This is probably the ultimate rejection, especially if she has high respect for you. Rejection of the act doesn't mean rejection of the person -- that should be explained to her. You can support her without necessarily giving approval of her request. A brief review of the present situation and a suggestion that there are other roads to follow night soften the blow. But don't play the role of her father or her mother.

4. Prescribe contraceptives and bill her family

This is another breach of confidentiality unless she and her family agree after proper counseling. Without that, this is not a rational option.

5. Prescribe contraceptives and charge her

While the charging of a child in this situation was condemned in the case of John, this case has a slightly different slant, and other things to consider. First, she is older (and may even have a job). Second, this is not the final visit; she will need to come back for refills of her prescription or for other care, so it is on-going. This point will have to be addressed when you have your chat with her. Certainly, necessary care for this first visit should not be refused because of the payment. Future care will have to be discussed -- and negotiated.

6. Prescribe contraceptives and forget about the bill

Depending on the circumstances, this may be the only viable alternative to conferencing with her and her parents, particularly if either party feels a strong emotional investment or blockade. I believe that the health professional should, if necessary, provide this first visit without charge. But that health professional does not owe continuing and repeated free visits, or continuing care without the parents' knowledge. Some arrangements would have to be made directly with the patient for handling this - both payment and parents.

Ethical Considerations

Although financial considerations do not drive this situation, they do occupy one niche in the problem. Once again, finances should never be the determining factor in the management of a patient. That is almost never in the best interest of the patient.

Here we are dealing with an older child--one perhaps mid-way between child and adult, that is, an adolescent. She has the hormones and the drive, as well as the uncertainties and vacillations of her age group. Plus, there are a number of other 16-year olds who are married. We have a situation that of necessity will be recurrent. Failure for her to obtain contraception will almost certainly lead to pregnancy. And that will almost certainly lead to family problems -- or worse.

This is a long-term situation, one in which the patient and her family will be embroiled for a long time. It is urgent that they get together sooner or later---better sooner--and reach an understanding. Do they want to try to curtail the sexual activity? Do they want to get counseling on sexual behavior for all of them? Do they want to ostracize her? Do they want to accept her behavior and look at potential pregnancy? Or what do they want?

Regardless of anything else, your initial role would be to sit down with her (standing consultations deliver the message of rush and indifference) and discuss the total situation. Confirm through your questions whether she really is sexually active (or merely planning to be). Explain the problems and the options. Getting contraceptives secretly is going behind her parents' backs and will eventually lead to confrontation. If you prescribe contraceptives, this act puts both of you in bad light with her family and perhaps with the community. She should understand that being sexually active always exposes her to unplanned pregnancy with its multiple repercussions.

Knowing she is street-smart, you know that the sexual behavior is apt to continue.

If she is just thinking of starting, counseling *might* help her hold off until a later age. Not too likely, but you might suggest it. Assure her that you are supportive of her but that the best route to follow is for her and her parents to sit together and discuss all the possibilities. Offer to sit with them as a buffer or, if that is uncomfortable for either of you, offer to get a counselor or other appropriate health professional to act as intermediary.

If she claims actual sexual experience, you should insist on a gynecological examination, including studies for Sexually Transmitted Diseases and AIDS for her protection, with the caveat that any positive findings would increase the urgency of consulting with her parents.

The health professional can be a fantastic intervenor and counselor -- if that health professional has the feeling and training to help. If not, he or she owes it to the patient and to the family to steer them to a health professional who can help.

Second Opinion

by Stanley Cohen, EdD
Vice Provost, Health Professions Division,
Nova Southeastern University
Professor and Chairman, Division of Medical
Humanities, NSU College of Osteopathic Medicine

I am especially pleased that factors other than purely medical ones are included in Dr. Melnick's analysis, because so often in actual practice the values of patients and their families are secondary to the physician's values. The resulting outcomes can be a disaster. Ignoring other influences such as ability to pay, family relationships and legal issues can result in decisions that may be medically correct but not right for the individual patient.

From a learning standpoint, the format in Lucille's case is really sound. The case is clearly presented, the options are comprehensive and the ethical analysis of each option is superbly outlined.

Let's take another look at the options.

1. Call her parents

Anyone who goes to a physician assumes that confidentiality is implied. Otherwise, when that trust is broken, the whole private relationship is broken. To assume that all young patients have a positive home environment and supportive parents is just plain naive. I once knew a father in my former counseling practice who almost physically killed his daughter when he discovered she was carrying condoms.

Lucille is coming to you for help as her physician. You are not her priest, rabbi or minister. That is not your expertise, but you are qualified to talk and listen to her without being judgmental. She also needs a thorough education on all aspects of her sexuality. Is she aware that the pill does not always work? Does she know the pill does not protect against HIV infection? Is she aware that "outercourse" is an alternative that some young people who are sexually active find enjoyable? Does she believe that refusing intercourse will result in loss of a boyfriend? Is her self-esteem so low that only her sexual activity can make her feel worthwhile?

I think Dr. Melnick is correct. Calling her parents will probably not change her behavior. It would probably be helpful to do the counseling with Lucille after the office is cleared out. It cannot be done in five minutes. Waiting until the office is closed does two things: First, ensures confidential dialogue because other patients and even staff would not hear what is shared; and second, you may need an hour or more to flush out all the thoughts and feelings, identify options, and look at the consequences of each option.

2. Refer her to Planned Parenthood

This option really worries me. My experience with some centers indicates that some personnel are not well trained to do Rogerian-type counseling which I believe works best with this type of case. Besides, referring her to a clinic does not relieve the physician of his or her responsibility to get her quality care, and in a way is a form of abandonment. She is your patient. Deal with it as a professional.

3. Tell her how disappointed you are in her

NO! NO! She already has enough negativity in her life to destroy her self-esteem. After all if she is sexually active and is asking for help to prevent pregnancy, she at least shows she is accepting responsibility for her behavior, and she ought to be told she has done the right thing in coming to see you. I would also let her know that asking you for help with a sexual problem is an O.K. thing to do. Teenagers may need permission to ask for this kind of help.

4. Prescribe contraceptives and bill her family

Billing the family has the same effect in violating confidentiality, autonomy, self-determination, and even violates the law in many states, such as Florida.

5. Prescribe contraceptives and charge her

While I would not turn her away without payment, I believe that some kind of minimal payment which she can afford would help her feel that she is earning your services even if that was fifty cents a week. Again, it helps to reinforce the notion of accepting responsibility.

Situation Three

Mary is 12 years old. Everything except her age is identical to the Lucille in Situation Two.

The Options

1. Call her parents.

2. Refer her to Planned Parenthood.

3. Tell her how disappointed you are in her.

4. Prescribe contraceptives and bill her family.

5. Prescribe contraceptives and charge her.

6. Prescribe contraceptives and forget about the bill.

A Look at the Options

1. Call her parents

The same confidentiality ethic should pertain here, even with a younger child. It becomes even more important when it shows the value of an on-going relationship between a physician or other health professional and a family. The fact that Mary had the courage at her age (and it takes courage) to visit you shows a significant strength of confidence.

You can utilize that in counseling this youngster and convincing her to talk to her parents or allow you to call them and invite them in for a discussion. It is not necessary to blurt out the entire story to the parents on the telephone, but a simple statement that Mary has a medical problem and we should sit down and talk about it. (But do not make an appointment for several weeks later, no matter how busy you are; this situation is urgent.).

The dangers of informing Mary's parents without her permission are even greater (because of her age) than what it would be in older children. You are the key player in this drama. True, you were pulled into it without warning, but as a physician, now that you are in it, you must follow through with help. Because of her age, it is almost an absolute necessity to include the family and there is far less rationale for you to prescribe without them.

2. Refer her to Planned Parenthood

This is a suitable alternative, if the patient refuses to allow you to call her parents. However, it should be explained to Mary as suggested for Lucille.

3, 4, and 5.

What was said for Lucille goes at least double for Mary. These are not viable alternatives.

6. Prescribe contraceptives and forget about the bill

While I have repeated the importance of not letting finances determine what you do -- or do not do -- this is a far less important factor with Mary. Her age makes most options relatively inoperable. The difficulty here is the first part of the option: Prescribe contraceptives. We must do everything humanly possible to save the family, that is, to get the patient and her parents together to solve what will be a lingering problem, and which needs all of their input.

Ethical Considerations

Our big problem here is the age of this girl. At twelve, no matter how mature or street-smart she seems, we are dealing with a less sophisticated, less informed, less mature patient. So, our ethical considerations become even more difficult: we are not only dealing with a dangerous situation, we are dealing with a girl far less able to handle it or make decisions.

This situation would challenge any family. Even the most highly functional family can be thrown into a tizzy -- although they may eventually adjust and "live happily ever after". But a less well-adjusted family may develop many dysfunctions as a result of this situation.

Therefore, there is need for extra emphasis and additional hard work on your part to convince her that her parents must become part of the solution. Mary must be made to understand that her parents must know, and they must aid her in meeting the challenge. And you must support her in this, even taking her part when necessary in the discussions in order to minimize hostility and retributions, and to keep the discussions on track.

A good starting point might be the need for a gynecological examination if she is indeed sexually active. Even children understand the need for an examination in a physician's office -- plus it can give you added ammunition for calling the parents.

One caveat I have already alluded to. In order to play the needed role in this situation, you should have a reasonable command of gynecology, and a fairly good grasp of adolescence and its problems. Otherwise, you become a relative amateur in a deadly serious situation. If you do not possess these tools, explain it to the patient and her family and then refer them properly. Until then, you are the pilot and cannot abandon them. You must be the go-between and try to eliminate or limit any harsh confrontations until you can refer the entire family to a competent gynecologist, psychologist or psychiatrist.

Second Opinion

by Stanley Cohen, EdD
Vice Provost, Health Professions Division,
Nova Southeastern University
Professor and Chairman, Division of Medical
Humanities, NSU College of Osteopathic Medicine

While this case is clearly stated, there is not enough information to make an adequate ethical judgment. Besides being a 12-year old, what is her sexual history? What is the age of the male or males involved? What age did she become sexually active, or is she still a virgin? Is her motivation to have sexual intercourse based on her desire to hold on to her boyfriend? What kind of pressure has he made on her? Does he threaten to leave her if she says no? Does she describe her relationship as one based on mutual love? Has she been exposed as a young child to pornographic materials such as videos or TVs? Does she have young female friends who are sexually active? Have drugs been involved with friends? If her male partner is an adult, Family Services needs to be advised since it is considered rape even with mutual consent.

1. Call her parents.

If, after much dialogue and urging, she says she cannot tell her parents, offer to make the call yourself. Offer to do this as her physician. You can do this with less threat to her. A decision of this magnitude made without guidance from a caring older person could result in tragic consequences. Don't allow this to happen.

Is it possible that Mary is being molested by her father, stepfather, mother's boyfriend, family friend, or other family member? In that case, Mary's reluctance to involve her parents may be more a function of fear of reprisal than fear of disappointing her parents. If Mary is being molested, you are ethically and legally obligated to inform the authorities. Mary's physical and emotional well-being is at risk without intervention.

2. Refer her to Planned Parenthood.

If she rules out all attempts to get her parents involved, then referral to Planned Parenthood is probably the next best option. However, even if she goes, the physician is still involved ethically. To assure Mary going, offer to make the appointment call to the center yourself. Ask her if she will allow Planned Parenthood to give you feedback.. Otherwise, your actions could be considered abandonment. Mary is still your patient and you are so responsible for care.

3. Tell her how disappointed you are in her.

Mary may have already lost much of her self-esteem. Doing this might compound the problem. Her values are her own. As a physician it is not your function to impose your values, unless she asks you. Try to understand her views through careful listening. Do less talking. Maintain eye contact throughout the dialogue. Give Mary your full attention -- you can do your chart notes later.

4 and 5. Prescribe contraceptives, and bill her family or charge her.

While it may be argued that she is too young to maintain confidentiality, the maturity level needs to be considered. If she has the level of intelligence to understand the implications of her decision, then to bill her family would violate the principle. In fact, in some states, this would even be illegal.

6. Prescribe contraceptives and forget about the bill.

If all of the above options are rejected, the only medically ethical decision is to prescribe contraception -- with the strong stipulation that she return with scheduled visits for physical checkups. It has been the tradition in medicine for many years to care for patients who need help without remuneration. Fees collected from this family over the years are sufficient without charging a 12-year-old for a few visits.

Situation Four

Billy is 8 years old. You have treated him over a number of years and have found him to be a difficult, obstreperous patient. This has caused family battles in your office. However, in the past few years, he has developed total confidence in you and has become cooperative. One day, driving past the local elementary school, you see Billy standing with some other children and smoking a cigarette. What do you do?

The Options

1. Call his parents immediately on returning to your office.

2. Stop and talk to Billy on the spot.

3. Wait till the next visit and ask to see him alone.

4. Do nothing; it's none of your business.

A Look at the Options

1. Call his parents immediately on returning to your office.

Remember always that Billy is your patient – not his parents nor the insurance company that is paying his bills. That carries with it a certain amount of confidentiality. If the situation implicitly meant immediate physical dangers to Billy or others, there *might* be a reason to call them. Barring that, calling his parents is a violation of the doctor-patient confidentiality.

Let's look at the situation. Until recently, Billy was difficult to manage in your office, so there might be an underlying dysfunction in family dynamics. That being said, reporting to them would possibly bring chaos, yelling, screaming, recriminations, physical punishment – any or all of them. Then, the question is: Will that do any good? Will that make Billy stop smoking? There is anecdotal evidence that it sometimes works and anecdotal evidence that other times it does not. Maybe most important, child-rearing experts would say that for the majority of cases this is not the constructive way to manage such a problem.

What harm would calling the parents do? If it destroys or even impinges on your relationship with Billy, it is dangerous. Billy might revolt and refuse to see you again as his physician, creating a problem for the family, and even more, making it necessary to find another physician. Then, he would have to develop confidence in that physician—something that it took a while to do with you.

If the family reaction were less severe – and you didn't lose him as a patient-- Billy might stay in your care but probably would never fully trust you again. You certainly would not expect him ever to tell you personal things (which might be necessary for his medical care). Would he take you into his confidence a few years later that he experimented with drugs and wanted your help or advice? Would he ask you about some "sexual" situation because he is confused by it? Hardly likely. And, even though it is difficult for all adolescents to confide in their doctors under such circumstances, a few will do it spontaneously, and some will talk on careful questioning. But only if the teen-ager has full confidence in the physician—and in Billy's case, that would be gone.

So, this is not a reasonable option.

2. Stop and talk to Billy on the spot.

Remember that Billy is with friends. We do not know whether they are smoking or not, but probably they are—as smoking has some social aspects.

In any case, what would Billy's reaction be? Remember again that he has in the past been a difficult patient and smoking is often a revolt against parents and society. Most likely, it would be embarrassment (in front of his friends, making the situation worse). Or maybe embarrassment because he had been showing off to his friends. He would become the laughing stock of his friends and all sorts of teasing would probably result. And you might look like a stupid adult. Since he has been hostile in the past, that embarrassment would immediately yield to anger. Predicting what his behavior would then be is difficult: he might challenge you, throw the cigarette at you, curse you, strike you—or the opposite: slither away, crying and completely crushed psychologically..

No one would expect him to extinguish the cigarette immediately and say, "You are right, doctor, I shouldn't be smoking and I'll never do it again." Yet, this is what this action is intending to do—that's the basis of stopping your car. And if he said that, you and he and his friends would know it was a lie.

This is not a solution.

3. Wait until the next visit and ask to see him alone.

This might be a logical approach. See him next time he is in your office and discuss the problem with him. On that first visit, Billy should be alone with you, and you should try to convince him to allow you to talk with him and his parents together. Then, you can be an intermediary and possibly prevent or reduce violent reactions. If he says OK, you can be the one to tell his parents what happened. You would introduce the subject in a calm and reasonable way, and maybe offer some suggestions. There should be no chastising and no preaching. You are trying to resolve a problem between child and family. If you are uncomfortable with this type of interview, you might even suggest referral to someone who handles this type of situation more than you do. Sounds reasonable, and the results might be what you want—but you must be prepared that it may not work at all.

Even in this option, there are inherent problems. The first thing you have to do is check your office to see when he is due for a visit. Billy may have been in your office last week, and not due for another year or so, or even six or more months. That's obviously too far from the incident to be of value.

Further, Billy is 8 years old, and if you are like most physicians, you will have his parents in the examining room with him. Thus, even if you could do this in a timely manner, you would have to say to the parents that you wanted to see Billy alone – or worse, lie to them about the reasons or make up a phony excuse for it. That would translate for Billy as a lie on the part of the doctor. What happens to confidence? Because of his age, this option becomes more difficult. This would work well if you regularly saw children alone for at least part of the visit— something we should all do when children reach about 11 years of age.

Probably the best choice in this kind of problem is somehow talking to Billy alone and then arranging for a child-parent-doctor conference. As you see, it is fraught with problems.

4. Do nothing; it's none of your business

First, you must decide whether it is your business or not. Your action (or inaction) may vary depending on that decision. If you really believe that you have no ethical obligation in this kind of situation, you will decide that it is not your business. Are you your brother's keeper?

It is important to note that this situation is a health matter, albeit long-term. That may help make the decision for you. But what if the incident you observed were gambling or fighting or destruction of property? Would that sway you? Is the ethics different? In effect, you would have to decide whether your "responsibility" or ethical involvement goes beyond health matters. If you think it does, you properly could be classed as a humanitarian—and that's good for a health professional. If you think not, you may just have tunnel vision—and still be a good doctor.

You probably do not have any obligation in this instance—certainly not any legal compulsion to intrude yourself. So why would you bother to do anything?

I think it's because most physicians really care about society and particularly about people and, more particularly, about individuals in potential danger. In spite of potential lawsuits (even in the face of "Good Samaritan" laws), many doctors will stop to help a stranger who has passed out, or to see what he/she can do in an automobile crash.

I also believe that most physicians would want to "do something" to help if he is their patient. What is ethical then? To maintain the doctor-patient relationship, to assist in some possible way and to alienate as few people as possible along the way. Most physicians would be uncomfortable for a long time if they did absolutely nothing for Billy.

I recommend that the reader return to Situation One and review the first two options, as so many of those statements apply to Billy's case.

Ethical Considerations

Billy's situation presents a number of complicating factors—making the ethical judgment more difficult for the physician.

First of all, the patient is in no immediate danger nor does this situation adversely affect those around him. So, there is no medical indication for interference. His life is not in danger. He is not going to get sick immediately (and that tells you that he has probably smoked before). No "medical" treatment is needed.

What you are dealing with is the beginning of a habit that eventually (40-50-60 years later) might create deadly disease—and you would like to prevent that. And so would his parents in all probability.

Further, Billy did not come to you with a "problem" that you could turn into a therapeutic situation. You are chasing the problem, making the situation more difficult.

Factors that might influence your thinking are many and include your relationship with the family. Are you close personal friends with the parents, or you are strictly occasional doctor-visit acquaintances? Are you a neighbor of the family and have a child of equal age (many implications)?

And above all, many competent and caring physicians might debate with themselves: Is this any of my business or am I just sticking my nose where it doesn't belong? What if he weren't your patient, but a child whom you know or you know his parents? Would you then feel any ethical compunctions? What if he weren't your patient but his parents were? What if he were just a neighbor's kid with no "professional medical" relationship to you. Now decide.

I have not discussed two of the most important questions that will influence both your decision and the outcome -- perhaps changing either or both to the extreme. Do YOU smoke? Does either PARENT (or an older sibling) smoke? I need not expand on the multiple machinations if either answer is affirmative. There is no more difficult conundrum than "Do as I say, not as I do." Even if there were a logical answer to that, it would be incomprehensible to an 8-year old. You would only be adding confusion to an already complex situation.

In this complicated drama of ethics, you must carefully choose what you can do best for this patient and the best choice for you. Then go with it. And hope. And hope. And hope.

Second Opinion

by Edward E. Packer, DO, FAAP, FACOP
Chairman, Department of Pediatrics
College of Osteopathic Medicine
Nova Southeastern University
Program Director, Pediatric Residency Program
Palms West Hospital

[Dr. Packer has combined his Second Opinions of Situation Four and Situation Five, and his comments appear at the end of Situation Five (page 44)].

Situation Five

Everything is identical to Situation Four

except that Billy is smoking marihuana

**[Please be sure to read Situation Four
before beginning this Situation]**

The Options

1. Call his parents immediately on returning to your office.

2. Stop and talk with Billy on the spot.

3. Wait until the next visit and ask to see him alone.

4. Do nothing; it's none of your business.

5. OR, call the police.

A Look at the Options

This situation concerns marihuana instead of a cigarette, so the face of this ethical problem changes considerably, even though it retains portions of the previous ethical considerations for the health professional. Because this now has legal aspects, it also becomes necessary to add a fifth option: Call the police.

1. Call his parents immediately on returning to you office.

Once again, there is consideration of the fact that Billy is your patient, with an on-going relationship. This must influence how you act, regardless of what you do. Hopefully, it will push you to try to help him as much as you can, within certain bounds.

There are several immediate considerations in this situation that were not present with the cigarette: First, it is a police matter. Second, he may incur illness from or reaction to the marihuana. Third, there is the possibility that he is likely to progress to a higher level of substance abuse if his behavior is not interrupted. Fourth, he may be friends with or consorting with the wrong people.

However, this is the same Billy who has familial dysfunction in his background or, at least, intrinsic behavior problems. Either of these may enhance the possibility of progression to stronger drugs. As before, notifying the parents as the primary answer to the problem, creates more potential damage. Parental over-reaction (which may follow being notified), or their interference or the imposition of restrictions will probably not do much toward correcting the situation. The harms described in calling the parents about smoking a cigarette are the same for marihuana, but probably more intensified. You must think of other or additional approaches.

The confidence that Billy has started to develop with you may be the only strong "handle" to rescue him from this situation. Anything that destroys or diminishes that confidence – like calling his parents outright—will totally eliminate the possibilities of rescue. I cannot over-emphasize Billy's need at this moment for a strong, supportive adult in his life.

There is even less reason here than in the cigarette incident to concern yourself with possible loss of Billy as a patient or even loss of the family as patients. Your personal equation regarding its effect on your practice, or income, must not enter into it.

Thus, calling his parents at once does not seem to be a viable option

2. Stop and talk to Billy on the spot.

As strong as the reasons are for not doing this when you see him smoking a cigarette, they are now so much stronger. Probably his reaction -- resentment and hostility-- would be considerably greater in this situation than in the last. Only harm -- to you and to Billy -- can come from this approach.

This is hardly an answer to the problem.

3. *Wait until the next visit and ask to see him alone.*

A mentioned before, the best choice in this kind of problem is somehow arranging to talk to Billy alone and then setting up a child-parent-doctor conference. Trying to do this is understandably fraught with dangers. It might work if the timing is right, but if you can work it out, the benefits are great.

Everything said in the cigarette situation is magnified here. There is no time to spare. Unless Billy is scheduled to visit your office within the next 7 days, you cannot wait and must find another solution. Obviously, there must be a meeting with Billy and his parents, either at once or within a couple of days (unless you are willing to drop the matter into the hands of the police or completely ignore what has happened). This will not wait until your first open appointment next month or whenever. It is an immediate must. If you are to be the "strong , supportive adult" in his life, you must find a way to do this, without creating waves of anger, mistrust and violence ahead of you. You must consider that it will take some of your time and create much stress for you, either way..

4. *Do nothing; it's none of your business.*

Either it is your business—as his physician, as an interested citizen, and as probably the only viable adult support presently in his life – or it's not. I believe that, ethically, it is your business, up to a point. Maybe like the adult being treated for depression until something more is needed. If you decide it is not your ethical responsibility, your alternatives seem to be "walking away" and making believe you never saw him smoking marihuana, calling the police immediately, notifying his parents at once or any combination of these. None are appealing, I would guess, to any physician, and most of us would be totally uncomfortable ethically in making one of those choices, it's tough to "let the chips fall where they may." Because this is also a legal matter, it adds a burden to your ethical decision.

Consider this: If he were hit by a car, you—any physician – would not hesitate to render immediate care and help, WITHOUT CALLING HIS PARENTS OR THE POLICE FIRST. As mentioned in the previous situation, most physicians would want to "do something" to help a young man in trouble—and you can be that helper.

5. Call the police.

Unless you are willing to "abandon" Billy or shirk any responsibility in this case, this cannot be a first choice. However, you must keep in the back of your mind that it could become – or might have to become -- a police matter at some point

Ethical Considerations

Billy's situation is now compounded. There are medical considerations, legal implications and increased psychosocial impacts. In taking any steps, you have a number of factors to consider: the extent of your involvement with Billy, your relationship with the parents and other siblings, degree of friendship between you and his parents, whether mother and father are also your neighbors or friends, and any relationships between your children and Billy.

You are his physician. He is in danger—immediate and long-term. Your ethical dilemma is: Are you going to help or not? If you decide to help—as most physicians would – what steps should you take?

I think you must find ways to work with the family and Billy to get him to stop using marihuana, stop associating with those who do, reconcile the family to avoid creating other family dysfunctions, institute preventive measures and conduct fair observation and follow-up.

First, you must evaluate this family. Is it so dysfunctional that this situation would be ignored or minimized (e.g., father smokes pot, mother shoots cocaine)? If so, maybe police and child welfare need to be involved. However, if they are an average family, the idea is to bring the family together ethically.

As their physician, you probably know best how they would react to various suggestions. I would, however, consider a plan like this. I would call the parents, and on some pretext, tell them that something in the child's record has caught your eye (a slight bending of the truth: his actions actually did catch your eye) and you think it important enough to talk with them, very soon, the next day or two (You must not let ANYTHING delay it longer than that.). Tell them to bring Billy along, as you want to check something. (You do. You want to find out how much he understands about what he is doing.)

On their arrival, request seeing Billy alone. Present the problem to him. (He may deny it—say it was the first time.) Explain the seriousness of the situation and tell him in strong tones that it is absolutely necessary for his parents to know. (Trying to work with Billy alone without his parents is treacherous and dangerous, and certainly not an option, especially at Billy's age.). Remind him that part of your desire is to keep him from being arrested. Stress that you will be "on his side," his support and protection when the family sits down together and that you will stand by him in every way possible to help him out of this morass.

Then, bring in the parents and explain the need for understanding, support and calmness. Sit down with the entire family and introduce the subject. It would be your job to keep the conversation level-headed (as difficult as it will be for the parents and maybe even for you), to prevent recriminations, insults, name calling, screaming, yelling or any of the other negative behaviors that would disrupt the goals.

Seek goals and closures. If you feel qualified to do psychotherapy – or to do "drug" counseling-- continue to meet with them and help them. If you do not feel completely comfortable with this role, or cannot spare the time, refer the family immediately to an appropriate mental health/ drug counseling professional or center – somewhere that he will get expeditious attention.

By being ethically involved, you may have just saved a life.

Second Opinion

by Edward E. Packer, DO, FAAP, FACOP
Chairman, Department of Pediatrics
College of Osteopathic Medicine
Nova Southeastern University
Program Director, Pediatric Residency Program
Palms West Hospital

I will offer a Second Opinion for Situation Four and Situation Five together since both pose some similar ethical questions. These scenarios represent closely related issues since smoking represents an important health hazard, substance abuse is associated with several important mental health issues and it is also illegal in most areas of the United States for a minor to posses or use either tobacco or marihuana.

The first principle to address is the role of the physician versus that of a private citizen. As physicians, we enter into a contractual relationship with a patient that is mutually understood and continues until a defined termination is established. Critical components of that relationship as stated in the American College of Physicians' ethics position paper, include tending to "the patient's welfare and best interests", advocating for the patient's health and access to health care, establishing a relationship of trust and mutual respect and protecting the confidentiality of a patient's health information.

Substance abuse, including tobacco use, represents an important hazard to the well-being of our patient, to whom we are committed to provide care. Marihuana use has the added concern of long-term mental health problems associated with its continued abuse. The American Academy of Pediatrics' position paper on substance abuse states that it is our responsibility to facilitate the assessment, intervention and treatment of children who use tobacco or marihuana. Yet, actual intervention is "required" only when this abuse has impacted academic, social or vocational functioning.

As the established physician for Billy in Situation Four and Situation Five, it is our duty to provide health care for this child. The use of these illicit materials places our patient at risk of several related health issues. Yet, Billy is a minor who legally cannot consent to his own health care and will require the assistance of his parents to provide transportation and financial support for any medical care that he receives. In order to treat Billy, his parents will need to participate at some level in his care.

The second principle to address is patient confidentiality. The child in these scenarios represents an established patient for whom confidentiality must be protected unless otherwise required by law. Physicians are not required to report substance abuse in any state, so confidentiality guidelines prevail with this patient. Further, the American Academy of Pediatrics stated in a 2002 policy statement that it is part of the "adolescent's bill of rights" to have protection from disclosure of medical information regarding mental health, sexual health or substance abuse issues. Please recognize that the term "adolescent" refers to the child's level of cognitive functioning and not to a fixed age. Physicians are mandated to disclose private health information regarding an adolescent only "if the physician suspects physical or sexual abuse of the minor" or "if the physician thinks that the minor poses a severe danger to him/herself or others" as stated in the American Academy of Pediatrics' position paper. *Confidentiality Issues in Adolescent Health Care.*

Both Situation Four and Situation Five pose a set of conflicting issues to the primary care physician: the responsibility to our patient's mental and physical health along with the requirement to preserve the child's confidentiality. Given this dilemma, the physician has very limited choices that are appropriate for this situation. First, if the child were to present to the office for any reason, it is both appropriate and endorsed by the American Academy of Pediatrics, to ask the parents for a private interview with the child. Information that the child discloses must be told to the parents only if it places the child or others in immediate or severe danger. Second, if the child were not to present in the near future, a letter could be sent to the family informing them that the child is due for a physical examination. If the family did not respond to your appointment request, a phone call could be made to the family encouraging them to have the child seen for an annual physical or further health care. A private discussion with the child could be attempted at this arranged visit. It is important that the physician is honest and professional with the child and his family at all times. If the physician loses the "moral high ground," then the family may not regard advice for this child's care with the required willingness and trust to take the necessary action. If the child is willing to discuss the abuse problem, then the physician can attempt to get the child enrolled into the appropriate mental health treatment program. Usually, mental health treatment will require parental participation for both permission to treat and financial support. Generally, children who agree to intervention will be willing to involve their parents providing the physician meets with the family to prevent an inappropriate response.

One potential outcome for these situations is that the child never presents for a visit or will not discuss the drug abuse problems with the physician. The physician risks compromising his/her professionalism and integrity by involving law enforcement or informing the parents without the agreement from the child. Some situations in the practice of medicine do not have the outcome that we would prefer as a physician. By always maintaining a careful ethical approach to all situations, the physician helps to insure that each patient care issue has the opportunity for the best possible result.

Situation Six

Agnes is an attractive 16-year old, the apple of her family's eye. She is an honor student, a valuable volunteer at the local hospital, the President of the Student Council, and she is strongly motivated to enter medicine. She comes into your office pregnant and insists that her sexual encounter was a one-time thing. What do you do?

The Options

1. Call her parents

2. Try to convince her to meet with you and her parents to discuss the possibilities.

3. Refer her to an abortion center.

4. Send her to her clergyman.

A Look at the Options

1. Call her parents.

All the admonitions in preceding cases about not calling parents as the first option apply to this young-lady-on-the-way-to-adulthood. Once again, the important considerations are confidentiality and privacy—especially important with a 16-year old.

We assume here, first of all, that the definite medical diagnosis of pregnancy has been made, one way or another. The expectation of this young lady in consulting you is obviously that she will get complete confidentiality; her visit implies that she has confidence in her physician. Thus, the first thing the physician must do is respect this confidence and support the patient.

From her stated history, she appears to be an intelligent young lady, and if she intended her parents to know, she would probably not have come to you first. Of course, the correct procedure is to ask her directly. If she says, "No," then she presumably has come to you for help to get out of a complex situation. Maybe she does or does not know her options. Perhaps she never considered notifying her parents as an option, or rejected it.

Even if you have strong feelings about including her parents. as most doctors would, there are several steps to start with before deciding to notify them: establish the presence of a pregnancy, explore her concerns and considerations, find out whether she wants her parents notified (now or maybe later) and explore her understanding of the situation. Not to do this is like prescribing treatment before hearing the complaint and examining the patient.

One additional factor must be considered. In some states, a female of any age becomes emancipated upon becoming pregnant. In other states, there is no emancipation, and in the remainder, there are varying degrees of "emancipation," including the necessity in some states of appearing before a judge for approval of the request without including the parents. In those granting full emancipation (Florida, for example, is one of them), the patient is free to make her own decisions without consulting or notifying her parents. In this situation, the physician may then ethically refer her for the abortion she wants. (Not that this is the most astute immediate action; some time should be spent reviewing the possibilities and ramifications with her before making any impulsive referral – to be sure that the young lady involved is making the best decision for herself.) Unless the physician knows and understands the actual law in his or her state, the best advice is for that physician to consult his personal lawyer immediately (this is an urgent situation).

All of these factors bear upon the ethical decisions of the physician.

2. *Try to convince her to meet with you and her parents to discuss the possibilities.*

Once you have established the base of information described above, this is probably the next—and best—step to take. Inherent in this situation are a number of factors---her desires, her parents' desires, family circumstances and dynamics, consideration of other siblings, good and bad points in completing the pregnancy, good and bad points in terminating the pregnancy, role of the baby's father, religious pressures, ethical pressures and vocational pressures. Those items do not include any legal implications that may be present or may add a positive or negative effect on everyone concerned.

To effect a solution in any matter when several parties are involved, probably the best first step is to get them to sit down together and discuss the possibilities, weigh them carefully and try to reach some agreement. This tense, dynamic, touchy and fragile kind of conference needs a steady and calm hand guiding it. That might be you as the physician or health professional. You must keep the meeting under control at all times, even before sitting down together, including not "sending her home to notify or talk with her parents."

To do this, you must be able, first, to spend the time necessary, and then to review all the possible ramifications and choices, without prejudice or "selling". Then, and only then, try to convince the young lady that she needs the help of her parents, and that they would probably want to be available to help her. If these conditions cannot be met by you, refer her (without making it sound or feel like a rejection) to a suitable agency, or to another health professional with great experience. Either one should be helpful, and open, with no preconceived notion of what to do.

So, it really comes down to three things: educating the patient about the consequences and choices; including of the rest of the family; and choosing between carrying to term or abortion.

3. Refer her to an abortion center

Before you make any referrals in one direction or another, you must ask yourself, "Am I the proper person to advise?" Do I have the qualifications and the experienced judgment to guide this young lady to a decision, especially if it's to be without her parents? If you have no background (training or experience), consider referral to a suitable, helpful, appropriate and balanced agency or other practitioner.

The decision for abortion actually should not be the doctor's decision, but the patient's, whether you are proceeding with or without the family. You may have strong feelings either way but they should not be imposed on a 16-year old. Like everyone else, a physician has the absolute right to have his or her own opinions on matters, his or her own mores and ethics. But the doctor does not have the right to impose those views on the patient and harangue the patient to do what the physician believes, either way. There are physicians on both sides of the abortion question, and fairness to the patient dictates that neither side should "sell" its viewpoint. You know: Do unto others.

If the ultimate decision is abortion, then a referral to an abortion center is in order, if you are not an obstetrician used to handling such cases. The center will be able to offer obstetrical evaluation, to perform the procedure (or have it performed) and to offer the necessary counseling. Most every female undergoing abortion needs some follow up—counseling advice, gynecological advice, contraceptive advice, or whatever is indicated by the status of the patient. If you as a health professional feel involved in any way (after all, she appeared in your office), you might consider personal follow-up to give the young lady continuity and support—and to help get her any other kind of support she may need—mental health therapy, family assistance or other.

If any of this is against your strong beliefs, DO NOT ABANDON the patient. You do not personally have to refer her to an abortion center, but you do have to see that she gets in supportive and capable hands for whatever is necessary. That may be .another physician, an agency, another health professional or a clergyman (see Option 4)—use your best judgment. The ethics involved is very clear: Above all else, you must, if possible, do the right thing (and the most helpful thing) for the patient.

4. Send her to her clergyman

Much of what was said in the previous option applies to this choice. Like abortion, it is one of the "options" available – not a *sine qua non*.

Once again, this is an apparent intelligent and sophisticated young lady. If she had a clergyman she could confide in—and wanted to – she would have consulted him. Perhaps she knew what her clergyman would say, and didn't want his/her advice – or didn't care. Instead, she sought the help and advice of a health professional.

If the young lady is desirous of seeing a clergyman, now or later, fine. She should see her clergyman or the family's clergyman or any clergy of her choosing. If she has no one of her own choosing, health professionals should try to help match up the patient with an appropriate clergyman, and perhaps offer several choices. The clergyman chosen should be the choice of the patient (and the religion of the patient).

However, this is an option if, after discussions called for above, she is willing to seek clerical advice, or really wants it. If so, that's what needs to be done. Undue persuasion, just as in referral to an abortion center, is not the purview of a health professional.

Ethical Considerations

This case is not simply a decision on abortion or carrying the baby to term, as it might appear at first blush. There are other ethical considerations.

> The wishes of the patient herself
> The family dynamics (suppose, as does happen, she had been sexually abused by her step-father)
> Role of the baby's father (suppose, as does happen, the father wants her either to have the child and will support it, or conversely wants her to have an abortion).

This is a complex situation involving a teen-ager who is pregnant and needs some medical care and guidance almost immediately. This is not a situation that can exist through a year of psychotherapy to get at the roots of any problem that might exist. Steps must be taken soon-- certainly medical/obstetrical processing. There is a family that must be considered and made aware before she starts to "show" or to have pregnancy symptoms. The "one-time thing" must be examined. Is it connected with bad family dynamics? Was it a hidden side of her personality? What is the role of the baby's father, now or later? What is the maturity level of the patient? How sophisticated is she? How responsible is she? Is there a "serious love affair" with the baby's father?

All this calls, not for the simple immediate decision of abortion or no abortion, but a careful examination of *all* the factors involved.

In any event, the ethical consideration is to do that which is in the best interests and desires of the patient, if at all possible—and maybe that's what we as health professionals should do. We should seek ways to achieve her desires without damaging others along the way or doing anything illegal.

Then, there is the ethical consideration of the health professional himself or herself. Are you knowledgeable enough to handle this—both medically and psychologically? Are you comfortable with handling such a situation? Do you really want to be involved? Ethically, if the answer is "No" to those—any of them—you must see that the patient gets into good and understanding hands before you let go. You might want to stay in the picture as an anchor, as a confidante, as a liaison to the family, or whatever role you might play to help the patient and the family. That is satisfactory also—as long as you do not interfere with the actual medical care of the patient once she is in capable hands.

This is a situation that, in almost all cases, will have an unsatisfactory course or ending for someone (patient, family, baby's father, society, the health professional) and that is to be expected because of the natural complexity, diametrical choices and strong feelings among so many people. As long as we accept that the ethics calls for doing the best thing for the *patient*, within societal and legal bounds, we are doing the right thing ethically.

Second Opinion

by Kenneth E. Johnson, DO, FACOOG
Associate Professor, Obstetrics/
Gynecology and Public Health
Director, Women's Health Center
College of Osteopathic Medicine
Nova Southeastern University

Introduction

Ethics plays a key role in Women's Health and the pregnancy of a minor like Agnes is always an intense and unfortunately common occurrence for physicians. Even more important is the medical reality that the practitioner not only accepts care for the mother but must be completely and ethically aware of the needs of the fetus. Ethics in the pregnancy of a minor like Agnes is about caring simultaneously for two patients and balancing the care for one to maximize the health outcome for the other. "If mom dies baby dies."

It goes without saying that in adolescent pregnancies like that of Agnes the minor is often unsure both of her desires about the pregnancy (abortion or keep the pregnancy) and her options. It is not uncommon for the patient to have supportive parents who intend to support the patient if her choice is to keep the child. On the other hand, if the patient is not in a supportive environment she may only be considering the abortion option.

The ethical approach to a pregnant minor begins with ensuring that the very first visit is a kind and caring one where the practitioner is open, nonjudgmental, and patient. Fortunately, in most states pregnant minors are emancipated so they essentially have the same rights as an adult and the practitioner can see and treat them without parental consent. This includes all the prenatal visits, the delivery and follow-up.

If the patient requests abortion after counseling, it is ethically essential to counsel on all the risks, benefits, potential side effects and alternatives. Even in the common event that the obstetrician doesn't perform abortions, he or she ethically should advocate for the patient by educating her on the medical aspects of the procedure. Critical in the discussion is the importance of seeking an experienced physician who offers abortion in a certified center.

It is also ethical and very important to discuss alternatives to abortion with minor patients including the option of delivering the baby and putting it up for adoption. Many couples legally seek out teenage mothers and make arrangements to adopt the child, giving the mother an additional option. Also there is the issue of abortion regret. Many women, and especially teenage mothers, abort and later have a deep sense of regret. Many studies say abortion regret approaches up to 80% of all mothers who choose abortion.

The ethical approach to a pregnant minor is not unlike the approach that should be taken with any woman or couple. Often there is time for the teenage mother to consider all her options. Effectively ensuring that the patient is presented all the available options is the ethical mandate. The intervention by a skilled, kind and compassionate physician can often play a major role in enhancing the outcome of what might otherwise be a very stressful situation.

Agnes

With specific respect to Agnes, I would make the following recommendations:

1. Because she is the "apple" of her family's eye, it is likely she has an excellent relationship with her family. If Agnes is comfortable letting them know what has happened to her, I always like to have the support of the family when working with a distressed minor. If Agnes decides to keep the pregnancy, it is likely her family will play a major support role not only during the pregnancy but for a long time afterward. In my career, I have personally enjoyed this scenario many times

2. If on the other hand, Agnes chooses not to have the family involved, I would recommend respecting her decision and help her in all areas of the decision-making process. Paramount is informing her of all the risks and benefits and alternatives of ALL her decisions. This, of course must be done in nonjudgmental language that Agnes can understand.

3. Certainly, if she admits to being spiritual, and I always inquire, I would encourage her to postpone any decision until after meeting with her choice of clergy. Interestingly, many physicians like myself are very spiritual and often pray with their

patients. If Agnes desired to pray with me — her physician — ethically this would be appropriate.

Situation Seven

This Situation is exactly the same as Situation Six, except that Agnes refuses to notify her parents, and says she will commit suicide if they find out.

[Please be sure to read Situation Six before beginning this Situation.]

The Options

1. Call her parents

2. Try to convince her to meet with you and her parents to discuss the possibilities.

3. Refer her to an abortion center.

4. Send her to her clergyman

A Look at the Options

Special considerations

With the threat of suicide, this situation takes on more significance, as both urgency and additional considerations complicate the situation – and they require special attention before delving into the specific options.

Any mention of suicide by an adolescent must be taken seriously, whether the health professional thinks that the patient is kidding around, or is treated by the teen-ager as a joke. The problem is that teen-age suicide is so ubiquitous and serious that every health professional must be aware of it and alert to its implications.

The third greatest cause of death in teen-agers, suicides occur 3000 to 5000 times a year, that is, 16 adolescent suicides a day. About 10% are in the 1- to 14-year old bracket. Important is that there are 15-20 gestures or attempts of suicide (such as Agnes) for each recorded one. Suicide and gestures make up about 12% of all emergency department visits and are most often unrecognized.

What bearing does this significant problem have on the health professional in this situation? Understanding the suicide problem and managing it become as important as the unwanted pregnancy—perhaps more so. Primarily, take the threat seriously. The situation becomes more charged, more urgent and more serious than before. The immediate handling? It is not "Oh, you're kidding," or "People who talk about suicide never do it" (a totally untrue myth; people who talk about suicide are contemplating it) or "You're just trying to frighten me into some action" or any such approaches. The real reply to the threat is one that shows understanding and concern, and invites further cooperation, such as "When people talk about suicide, it means they are unhappy. How can I help you?"

Ignoring or pooh-poohing the threat is like ignoring or laughing at the patient who is waving a gun.

This serious additional problem creates a more complex ethical situation than before. What would the responsibility be for a health professional faced with a suicide threat, even without the complication of an unwanted pregnancy?

Walk away from the entire matter? This would be abandoning the patient, a moral and ethical calamity, and something probably no physician would do.

Do psychological/psychiatric counseling? This is a consideration, provided you are qualified. Without background and experience in these matters, this would be a dastardly thing to do—and few professionals would attempt it.

Refer the patient to an appropriate mental health professional or center or suicide prevention program? This appears to be the only viable ethical and professional choice. But there is a problem: You still haven't done anything, one way or the other, about the pregnancy problem. And both problems are urgent and compelling—they cannot wait for prolonged therapy.

Now let's look at the options as originally presented for Agnes.

1. Call her parents.

Two ethical problems now exist: an unwanted pregnancy and a suicide threat. And we have a seemingly mature and apparently sophisticated 16-year old who appears to be capable of making her own decisions. But notice the "weasel" adjectives: "seemingly" and "apparently". Beware! There is always a possibility that she cannot make the necessary decisions!

For either the suicide threat or the unwanted pregnancy, this option does not seem to be a live one. Immediate notification of the parents is probably not in the best interest of the patient, and that is the major consideration in this ethical discussion. It may be unethical at this point, although it must be apparent that sooner or later they must be told or would find out.

One of the few ethical breaches of privacy or confidentiality in the field of psychiatry (and it is usually explained to the patients) is the obligation of the physician to report any realistic threat to the patent herself or to others. Under these ethical guidelines, you might feel justified in notifying her parents, particularly if you feel that the threat is realistic – after, of course, discussing the situation in its entirety with the patient. This is truly a dilemma.

I believe that notifying parents at this stage would be an ethical error. First, it violates the doctor-patient confidentiality. Second is the cloud of the suicide threat – she might kill herself if they find out (or before they do). And she might. So this option is not practical to me.

2. Try to convince her to meet with you and her parents to discuss the possibilities,

All ethical consideration – and practical ones, too – point in this direction. What would be better, given the two unmoving clouds that hang over the situation, than to have the family sit together under carefully controlled conditions and talk over the problems? Together, they might reach a mutually agreeable solution, with guidance from a skilled health professional—you or a mental health person you recommend.

This focuses on the best management of the two problems. But you, the health professional, must guide, beg, cajole, plead—in multiple meetings in a short period of time — with the parties to enter this phase, especially Agnes. This will take almost superhuman skills. Maybe this is something you have no training for or no heart to do, since it implies a commitment of time, an expenditure of effort and a strong dedication. If you have the training and skills, go to it. If not, get an immediate and urgent referral to an appropriate specialist.

3. Refer her to an abortion center.

Yes and No.

Yes, if that is the only way Agnes will allow you to include her parents in the discussion. Good abortion clinics make sure the patients get good counseling and, I hope, even offer the opportunity *not* to have an abortion—something that might ease the anxiety of some parents. They also are experienced with women whose pregnancy situations lead them, too, to consider suicide. So this may be the best approach available to un-muddle this situation.

No, if the referral is merely to get Agnes an abortion (without her parents knowing about it) or to get the case "off your back."

4. *Refer her to her clergyman.*

This is a viable option if either the patient or parents express a desire for it. There is much good that can come from such a consultation in certain situations, but it carries much trouble if imposed on the parties.

Ethical Consideration

Everything detailed in the ethical considerations for Agnes in the previous instance apply to this situation. With the threat of suicide, these may carry more impact and ramifications than before.

The ethical principle that is so important here is that we are obligated to do that which is best, or most helpful, for the patient—while doing nothing illegal, yet maintaining damage control, that is, keeping harm and hurt to others at a minimum. (In this type of situation, however, there is inherent damage and agony whatever way it may be settled.)

The striking dilemma connected with this suicide threat is whether to violate the patient-doctor confidentiality and call the parents or to maintain that privacy until further resolution of the case. Only the physician sitting with the patient can (and is obligated to) resolve this question. And it is almost impossible to second-guess it, depending on the outcome.

This case cannot be distilled down to abortion versus non-abortion or to minimizing a suicide threat. Each problem aggravates the other and adds previously unexpected ethical problems. To get through this morass of ethical problems will take, from everyone: patience, consideration for others, time, planning, calmness, equanimity, adult thinking and a few dozen other attributes. It is a difficult, almost insurmountable task at best.

But with some of those needed characteristics and a dedicated health professional "steering the ship", much can be done to minimize the problems and keep the family intact -- while doing the best possible thing for the patient.

Second Opinion

by Kenneth E. Johnson, DO, FACOOG
Associate Professor, Obstetrics/
Gynecology and Public Health
Director, Women's Health Center
College of Osteopathic Medicine
Nova Southeastern University

[Please be sure to read the Introduction to Dr. Johnson's Second Opinion for the previous Situation]

Suicide in adolescents in epidemic in America and therefore must be taken very seriously. In the case of Agnes, her unintended pregnancy makes the possibility that she would attempt to harm herself much more likely. Considering the increased complexity of her case with the addition of the threat of suicide, a multidisciplinary approach is often the most effective. For this very real and intense situation for Agnes, I would recommend the following three approaches:

1. First, I would assure Agnes that a team of support personnel, including myself as the leader, will guide her through this situation and we will never "give up" on her, regardless of whether or not she allows me to notify her parents.

2. I would then carefully try to assess why Agnes feels that suicide would be a suitable option, and

hope that with kindness and concern she would begin to see the futility of this option. If she begins to trust me and the suicide threat proves only to be a "call for help," I would do just that—help and support her, as I previously mentioned.

3. If Agnes convinces me that she is suicidal, I would not hesitate to Baker Act her and insure her proper and complete treatment. It is likely in this situation that her parents would eventually be notified and social support would be provided as needed.

   In the end, we must do what is best for mom and baby.

Situation Eight

There is a case of hepatitis in the camp bunk of Charles, age 7. His mother refuses immune globulin The next week, she brings him to your office for a school physical and, in front of Charles, asks you to write a note that you have given him hepatitis immunization, so that he can go to class. What do you do?

The Options

1. Give her the note because she has a large family and you care for many of the children.

2. Refuse to write the note

3. Tell her next time not to ask in front of the child.

4. Explain the "facts" to her and ask her to seek another physician to care for Charles.

A Look at the Options

1. Give her the note because she has a large family and you care for many of the children.

This is probably the worst option you can exercise. Not only is it unethical, it is immoral and illegal. As indicated several times before, considerations by the doctor that are based solely, or mainly, upon economics or upon the doctor's income are totally unethical. To do something this egregious, just for considerations of practice or money, is inconceivable, although I have known instances of similar situations where decisions were made on this basis.

Aside from the monetary aspects, there are the legal implications. Issuing a false document (such as writing the note) would be, at least, misrepresentation but at worst might be a felony, which calls for possible jail time. What penalty might result depends on the exact circumstances and the applicable state laws. In addition, there is possible action by the appropriate state examining board -- every possibility up to and including loss of license. While legalities are not the purview of this book, certainly anything that is illegal is also unethical -- automatically.

To me, this is absolutely an ethical no-no.

2. Refuse to write the note.

This is one of the most viable options, because such an untrue note should never be written. However, the manner in which the refusal is made is important from both a humane and ethical standpoint.

I think it would be cruel, as well as unethical, to make this refusal in front of the child. Doing so, would require the physician to explain to the mother that this would be an out-and-out lie or some similar explanation. This would, in the eyes of the child, indict the mother as a liar. It is not the physician's place, ethically or otherwise, to do this. So the refusal should *not* be done in front of the child nor should an explanation of its immorality.

The only way to do this in an ethical manner would be to ask the child to wait in another room while you review things with his mother, or take the mother into another room. At that time, you can explain to the mother the problems with your issuing a false statement, as well as pointing out the impact on Charles of a collusive lie between physician and mother. Then you should refuse in a polite, non-insulting manner and you can bring the entire matter to a close.

One other consideration might come into play. You should also explain to the mother the public health aspects, the effect on other children of a physician offering a false note about immunization. You might even expressly say that if this happened with a number of his classmates, the community would fail to be immunized and that would make her son more susceptible to getting hepatitis.

So, from any angle, this is not a viable solution and should not be used alone under any circumstances.

3. Tell her next time not to ask in front of the child.

Regardless of what option or solution you choose. there is one thing that should be pointed out to the mother. Make clear that asking the doctor to lie, in front of the child, not only makes his mother a liar, and his doctor a liar, but will eventually weaken his trust in both of them. And, obviously, this benefits no one – and can be quite harmful.

It also matters where you tell the mother this. If you say it in front of the child, you are emphasizing her dishonesty and perhaps creating in the child a sense that, under some circumstances, it is acceptable to tell a lie. It should be told to the mother in the absence of the child so that there is no disturbance to the mother-child relationship or the child's confidence in you as a physician.

4. Explain the "facts" to her and ask her to seek another physician to care for Charles.

This is a slightly different option from the last ones. If you choose this one, again it must be done in the absence of the child for similar reasons. You must emphasize the unethical, the immoral and possibly illegal aspects of her request without degrading her (in itself an unethical act), as well as its impact on the public health (which includes her child).

As in any untenable situation, the physician always has the right (ethically, morally and legally) to dismiss the patient from his practice, provided he continues to care for the patient until that patient is able to get another physician or until a reasonable period of time has passed. While I believe that the doctor should refuse (in some way) the mother's request for a false certificate, I personally would also dismiss the patient from my practice. It certainly would weaken all my dealings with the patient's mother in the future, as I would be suspicious about things she told me. Can I believe her description of symptoms? Can I believe her request for a particular change of therapy? Or anything? My trust in the veracity of the patient's mother is destroyed. Therefore. I would not want to take care of the child, as much as I might like him, because of possible potential harm to him through mother's untruthfulness.

I realize that not every physician might feel this strongly about the situation. But I do. Once again, the ethical choice is up to the individual physician – depending on what he or she can live with or cannot live with.

Ethical Considerations

This situation illustrates the role of lying in ethical considerations. I realize there are, or may be, situations in which it may seem right to tell a lie to protect the patient -- either for maintaining privacy or for some special consideration. But for any other reasons, a lie is not acceptable as ethical, whether it is done for the "convenience" of a patient (or of the physician), for monetary reasons, or for anything else. There is an old philosophy that if you do not tell a lie you never have to remember what you said. Analogously, in such situations as this, if you do not lie, you never have to look over your shoulder at any time for possible repercussions.

In situations such as this one, legality also comes into play, complicating the problem, and adding to it the ethical considerations of committing an illegal act.

In addition, the role of public health is important. Public health agencies have as their responsibility the protection of the public in all health matters. Therefore, they would certainly have a strong interest is such a situation and may even be required to take some action, up to and including legal action.

Much of the ethical considerations needed in this type of situation will already have been established within the physician's personality and, in general, he or she will act almost reflexly. Situations like this do not usually require long periods of agonizing self-examination on ethical involvement on the doctor's part.

Care should be taken to express clearly to the mother two things: first, your discomfort with being asked to write a falsehood, and second, the negative aspects, as it affects your relationship with her, the child's impression of the situation, public health or your continuance with his care. And none of this needs to be done in a hostile or angry mode but should be carried out in a quiet and orderly manner. Losing your temper, showing anger, or raising your voice may create an emotional reaction in the mother, making it difficult for her to accept the pertinent facts that you have presented. (Such action as this on your part may itself be intrinsically unethical.) Rather, you should present them as facts, and only facts, whether you keep the patient or dismiss the patient.

If you decide to have the patient placed under another doctor's care, you should explain to the child something that he will understand about why you refused to do the note, and why you are sending him to another physician. Make sure that the child does not feel he has done something wrong, thus creating this situation. Children often feel that a problem is something they caused, and it may be necessary to reassure the patient -- maybe several times, and rather strongly -- that nothing in this situation is his fault. Perhaps, something like blaming it on an incompatibility between the personalities of you and the mother (which it really is), but not by calling the mother a liar or indicating that she asked you to do something false. The child may even put the facts together for himself and recognize what is happening. What you do not want to do is destroy the mutual confidence between the mother and child while accomplishing what might be best for the patient, and even for you.

Second Opinion

by Frank DePiano, PhD
Vice President for Academic Affairs
Founding Dean, Center for Psychological Studies
Nova Southeastern University

Struggling through choices between two conflicting values is simultaneously difficult and essential for development of good moral character. In this case, the doctor is struggling with the need to be honest and forthright on the one hand, while maintaining the sense of esteem a 7-year old has for his mother on the other. Also at stake is the rapport between the doctor and, in this case, the mother and child patients.

As stated in opinion one, the first option of complying with the mother's request for the doctor to lie, is no real option at all. It is simply wrong, morally, ethically and legally for the doctor to falsely report a medical intervention. So let's put this choice in the category of "Never do this" and look at the two more viable options.

The doctor, in front of the child, explains to the mother that she is asking him to lie and denies the request, versus, *excusing the child and, alone with the mother, declining the mother's request for the doctor to lie.*

The most compelling concern expressed in opinion one is that the mother–child trust may be harmed by questioning the mother in front of the child. Therefore, the child should be excused and the doctor should confront the mother alone. There also are several down-sides to this approach. Maintaining the mother-child relationship is given primary consideration in the first opinion and is absolutely important to consider. Certainly, if the physician clumsily confronts the mother, embarrassing her or diminishing her value in the eyes of the child, the best interest of the patient(s) is not served. If, in fact, the confrontation is handled in such a clumsy way as to cause a long-term problem between the mother and child, an actual ethical violation may occur and I personally would consider the doctor to be negligent.

Let's look at this option in another light, however. How does a child develop a sense of morality, a concern to do what is ethical, or a drive to choose what is right versus wrong? Usually moral development requires a great deal of nurturing and fortitude. For this type of moral conduct to develop, three conditions are generally necessary. First, knowledge of what is ethical or moral must occur. This knowledge can be acquired through a variety of methods and is beyond the scope of this discussion. Second, the ethical/moral behavior needs to be observed. This allows both the general behavior itself to be understood as well as the subtleties associated with a complex ethical behavior to be learned. Third, once the child attempts such ethical behavior, even if the behavior itself only approximates the desired behavior, the child needs to be praised and recognized for her/his behavior.

In the case presented, certainly there is risk associated with discussing, in front of the child, the implications of the mother's request to falsely certify an inoculation. To be sure, a clumsy and an insensitive approach would likely destroy the doctor-patient relationship and could have a detrimental effect on the mother-child relationship. But, like so much of a doctor's work, all aspects of it, it requires a great deal of skill, sensitivity and good judgment. In this light, a sensitive approach in which the implications of the request are discussed with the mother, and in which the child is allowed to observe and participate in the discussion, may well provide the child with a) a rudimentary understanding of the ethics involved in this particular situation, b) modeling of the doctor and mother working through the ethical dilemma, c) first-hand observation of the difficulties associated with adhering to ethical standards and d) an observation of how two caring and respected adults work through an ethical problem.

This skillful and perhaps time-consuming intervention may go a long way in fostering the moral development of the child. Since this development is not automatic but rather learned and nurtured, it is too important an opportunity to miss by simply dismissing the child and completing the discussion with the mother in the absence of the child.

Situation Nine

George Roberts is a 5-year old with severe kidney failure and is on intermittent dialysis. Getting a kidney appears to be extremely difficult. Mrs. Roberts seeks your advice. She wants to become pregnant immediately, have an abortion at six months and transplant a kidney from the fetus to save the life of her one and only beloved son. What do you do?

The Options

1. Tell her it's a good idea.

2. Tell her it's a bad idea and talk her out of it.

3. Discuss the procedures involved and the ethics of all of them.

4. Counsel – Consult -- Conference

A Look at the Options

1. Tell her it's a good idea.

Even though a first hearing might lead some persons to utter such a comment, any real thinking will make us realize that it is dangerous to respond impulsively to such a deadly serious proposal. An immediate conclusion is dangerous — in spite of the fact that a person's first thought or impulse is said to be the right one in many instances.

What makes it a bad idea is that such a procedure may also destroy the life of the second child, leaving the mother with no children at all. Her lack of full understanding may have led her to grasp at what appears to be an easy solution. But the physician must spell out all the dreaded possibilities.

This is not a good option, ethically or otherwise.

2. Tell her it's a bad idea and try to talk her out of it.

This is the other side of the coin, but the reasoning against impulsive conclusions holds here too. Without previous experience (and who has any great experience with this specific problem?), reaching a logical opinion might take labored thinking and time.

It does not appear to be a good option.

3. Discuss the procedures involved and the ethics of them all.

There is no question but that the very first step should be for the patient to understand the ramifications of her suggestion. Perhaps she has insufficient information. Perhaps she has not processed the information properly. Perhaps someone else is trying unduly to influence her. Whatever the situation, she must learn all the facts, values and dangers -- in advance. Without them, she cannot really begin making a decision.

Maybe your starting point should be first to support her, as "I know the difficulties you are going through and I'm sure you've thought a great deal about solutions. I'm here to help you in any way I can. First, tell me what you know about your plan and why you are seeking it."

Be sure she understands all the ramifications — medical, psychological and social — both bad and good. You must make clear the dangers to the fetus, up to and including death. You must emphasize the potential handicap to the fetus if it lives, that is, living with one kidney and the danger it creates if kidney disease occurs. Be sure to include the psychological impact on George, knowing for a lifetime about the death or impairment of his "brother or sister," as well as this mental trauma to the rest of the family..

Once again, the ethical approach is *not* to decide for the patient but to offer all the information you can and then help the patient decide what *she* wants to do. Whatever your personal feelings and beliefs, you must not impose them on her, even though it is your prerogative, after reviewing with her all the possibilities, to express your preferences – not "sell" them, but express them.

Since most of the alternatives have ethical implications, these should be explained to her so she understands them clearly. Inquire about her ethical feelings or religious beliefs or moral standards, or absence of them. Whatever those feelings are, she most likely will have some emotional attachment or rejection toward many of the choices. So you must make the implications clear to her.

4. Consult—Counsel—Conference.

Not many physicians are rounded enough to provide all the information needed. For me, I would want to consult with her son's nephrologist (about the boy's condition and the implications of the mother's desire), a competent neonatologist, a psychiatrist (regarding the mother), a child psychiatrist (about the effect on the patient), and a well-grounded ethicist. Therein lies the complexity of the situation.

Ethically, can you – or any one person—have the credentials to put together sound advice? For, after all, once you have those consultations, it is necessary to conference with the mother (and father?) and then counsel them – once more bringing together the best advice you have gathered.

Perhaps the most ethical thing—and the most helpful thing—and the most practical thing—would be to refer the patient to a center that offers all of those services to help her. Sometimes the most ethical approach is to give up the case to a more experienced provider.

To repeat, ethics is doing the right thing for the *patient*, hurting as few others as possible and not conflicting with society or the legal system. In this instance, who is the *patient*—the mother or Charles?

So it would seem that the most ethical approach is to learn what the mother knows, include the father, consult with necessary authorities and then counsel the mother (and father?). Even if you give up control of the case or stop being "captain of the ship," you, as the primary physician, can continue to support the entire family psychologically -- as an advisor or in any way possible, whatever path she chooses. That would add great ethical impact to resolving this exasperating situation.

Ethical Considerations

This is a highly anxious, emotionally-charged, confusing situation, requiring from you an almost-immediate reaction of some sort. You have a desperate mother, grabbing for some solution to save her son's life. How will you help?

As we indicated in the discussion of the options, this is not the spot for impulsive recommendations or snap decisions or top-of-the-head advice. This complex puzzle must have carefully thought-out inquiries and solutions.

Your immediate reaction – that is, the very first words you say -- should be to let her know you recognize her anger and desperation and that you are available to try to help her. Any other action is premature.

Ethically, you will have to decide how much you can help her or will help her. You have to decide whether your medical knowledge is sufficient to carry through completely, or whether you want to continue, or whether additional help is needed. So, you first let kindness, consideration and concern shine through, so she realizes that you are on her side, regardless of what else you suggest.

Having done that, your ethical options appear to be, first, gently to "wash your hands" (whatever your reasons) of the problem by suggesting immediate referral to an appropriate person or center—a transplant center, a counselor who deals in these matters, or the like. The other option at this point, ethically, is to start as you would with any medical complaint—take a history. She must understand that you cannot recommend any action or further help until you know as much of the background as possible.

If you are not fully cognizant of George's medical condition, first obtain full and accurate information about him. If, on the other hand, you are aware of her son's status, you will want to know at least several other things: What does she think her idea involves? Does she know the advantages and dangers involved? Is her husband part of her request, or opposed to it, or an agreeable partner? Has she already looked into any aspects of the plan? How strong are her feelings about it—or is she merely offering this in desperation, hoping that someone will offer something better? Plus any ancillary information you can elicit.

Here is another fork in the road. One fork, if you decide you are capable of managing this (possibly with some additional consultations), is to start making necessary arrangements. The other fork, if you decide you cannot, or do not want to, handle this, is to make immediate (not sometime next week or whenever someone gets around to it!) inquiries or contacts to get her the best possible advice, so she can make up her mind.

Either way, you will have treated the mother ethically and hopefully contributed to some solution to her problem.

While deliberately downplayed to simplify the complexity, serious attention must be given to the role of the husband, the patient's father. For he is an important player, and must be considered, must be consulted, and probably -- both in an ethical and legal sense-- must be part of the decision-making process. However, because of the pressures, you cannot wait to start the immediate reactions as described here. Including the father calls for meeting with both him and mother very (that's *very*) soon and follow the course outlined, with the two of them.

If there are marital problems—separation, divorce, strained relations—ethics would dictate the inclusion of a marital counselor or other professional with experience in cases such as this.

You should also take cognizance of any strong religious feelings, or other moral suasion, that might affect the recommendations or course of action. This, too, must be done early.

Neither the human actions nor the ethics in this situation are easy or simple. It takes super effort (and lots of time), and in the long run, even if everything is done to resolve it in the best of conditions, there may still be some unhappy people.

Second Opinion

by Robert Locke, DO, FACOP
Division of Neonatology
Clinical Associate Professor of Pediatrics
Christiana Hospital/ A. I. DuPont
Hospital for Children
Thomas Jefferson University/School of Medicine

Maternal love, instinct and the will to protect and ensure the life of her child can often lead to creative and interesting situations. This mother's medical proposal is neither legal under United States law nor is it medically feasible. Although the ethical situation created by her proposal appears straightforward, it is not. Similarly, it is not an uncommon ethical scenario.

Conceiving and bearing a child for the specific purpose of creating a compatible hematopoetic stem cell transplant has already been undertaken with success in this country. Indeed, physicians and allied health care workers have already been sued for failure to advise parents of this option to save a family member, an event symbolic of the legal system's ability to outpace and even stymie adequate public ethical debate.

Although the creation of life for the specific purpose of histocompatible stem cell donor is not without its own ethical ramifications, the scenario under discussion is somewhat different, at least on the surface, from the case of George Roberts. Stem cells can be obtained from the placenta-cord blood after delivery without harming the newborn. In contrast, in the hypothetical situation posited here, the mother is planning for a late abortion in the hope that fetal kidney will be transplanted to her 5-year old son. The medical success of such an undertaking is unlikely to yield a successful transplant outcome. The fact that this is not a viable medical option in terms of transplant success will be temporarily ignored for the next portion of the ethical discussion, as this may not be true for other fetal organ tissues and may change with time. The ethical parameters surrounding this mother's request deserve further exploration, however.

Major transplant and related societies have rejected the concept that a person should be produced or created for the specific purpose of tissue or organ donation. These statements, as outlined in ethical guidelines, arise out of concern for respect of the personhood of the fetus and the concern for potential compromise of free-will and/or coercion in the reproductive decision-making of mother. In addition, under US federal law (NIH Revitalization Act of 1993; Public Law 103-43, sec.112), the use of fetal tissue obtained for the specific purposes of directed transplantation to a specific donor regardless of the source of funding is prohibited. The ethical issues are intertwined with autonomy and concern over who the patient is. Is it the mother, the 5-year old child, the fetus, or all three? Most importantly, all of these issues, ethical viewpoints and laws are further clouded by the abortion debate.

Mothers can electively, and in practice, legally obtain an abortion before fetal age viability. Recent bills introduced into Congress and placed before the Supreme Court to limit abortion have failed on an ethical and legal basis if they do not protect a mother's right to obtain an abortion on medical grounds. Even if one objects to the abortion, what is the situation if the mother obtains an abortion as is currently allowed? Is it ethical not to use the fetal tissues to save the life of another individual, if medically possible? Is it wrong to deprive the 5-year old child of life-saving organs once the fetus is already aborted, assuming the hypothetical situation in which the procedure could be successful? Should we deny the life of the son to protect the fetus? Would it be more or less ethical if the aborted fetal tissues were donated to the designated recipient, the mother's 5-yr old son, or a random recipient? How do we as physicians/health care workers balance the ethical interests of society, the mother who came to us as a patient, her 5-year old son, and the potential life of the fetus? What if the mother stated that she wanted to use pre-implantation genetic diagnosis to identify two embryos, and sacrifice one of the twins to save her other child? In that scenario, she would have two live children, whereas if she chose to do nothing, then her only child would die. What is the ethical morality of permitting one life to perish to save the potential of another?

It is possible, as explained above, to create life for the specific purpose of creating hematopoietic stem cells for a designated recipient, usually another family member. The fetus is allowed to grow to term and the cord blood is used. This scenario appears different from the mother who plans to have an abortion and use the fetal tissue, but the lines between the situations are not well defined. To obtain a histocompatible stem cell match, many embryos are created by in-vitro fertilization and then tested by pre-implantation methods to selectively obtain the embryo that is a match. Only that embryo is implanted. What happens to the other embryos that are stored or eventually destroyed? Many conceptions-implantations-pregnancies do not carry to the point of viability. What is the ethical difference between a conception that occurs in this fashion and results in a miscarriage or fetal loss in the second trimester and the mother in this case-study who wants to create life and terminate? All of this depends upon whether life is viewed as starting at conception or at birth. If life is considered to begin at conception, there is no significant difference. If life is thought to begin at the moment of birth, then there is a difference.

These are ethical issues that need to be debated and determined by society, rather than by individual physicians on a case-by-case basis. Although these issues have been partially addressed by transplant committees, an ethical resolution remains unclear. There is mixed support for the statement by the American Society of Transplantation Surgeons prohibiting the creation of life for the specific purposes of designation of organs and tissues for transplant. An NIH panel convened to address transplant issues, which supported the above AST statement, also suggested that if there is an insufficient supply of transplant organs, this issue should be readdressed. This is the situation in this hypothetical case scenario. The mother was motivated because of the lack of a suitable organ donor for her son. Survey research in Canada also displays some equivocality about this issue, in which only a slight majority favors such a restriction, with the remainder divided between permissible and undecided.

In this specific case situation, the correct ethical actions are options #3 and #4, which are to discuss, counsel, conference, and maintain a dialogue. We are presented with a mother desperate to save the life of her son. What she is really asking for is help -- help for her son, help for her family, and potentially, help in accepting an end-of-life situation. Outright rejection or acceptance of her initiative is neither a viable option nor does it meet the medical needs of the mother or her family. Listening, sympathizing and including the family as partners will open the door for optimizing medical care, permit greater understanding of medical decision-making and limitations by the family and allow her family's health care team the best opportunity to meet their needs. This should not occur in isolation. A team approach and open, bi-directional, honest conversations between family and the multitude of health care workers involved in the care of complex situations has always been an essential foundation of appropriate health care. Family participation, open sharing, individualization of care and thoughtful reflection are essential to the ethical implementation of health services, even when the final result is not exactly what a family desires.

Thus we have seen that there are three distinct and partially competing ethical pathways that need to be engaged simultaneously. One, the creation and termination of a pregnancy for the purpose of directed donation of fetal organs for a specific recipient is incompatible with normally accepted guidelines for ethical decision-making. Two, individualization of life-death decision allows for the potential optimization of ethical choices in unusual situations. Three, maintaining a dialogue between health care providers and patients is an ethical obligation within itself.

Situation Ten

You are a physician who has constantly expressed strong feelings against abortion. This has brought you into conflict publicly with a number of staff members at your hospital. Your 13-year daughter is raped by a 16-year old mentally defective boy, and now is pregnant. What would you do?

The Options

1. Send her "away to school" for a year..

2. Arrange for an abortion for her.

3. Accept the pregnancy and arrange for an adoption.

A Look at the Options

Unlike some of the other situations, this one presents a clear-cut dilemma. Whatever way you look at it, a decision has to be made either to abort the child (with all the resultant hullabaloo) OR let the child go to term and then keep the baby or send the baby for adoption. Therein lies the wrenching, but realistic drama.

1. Send her "away to school" for a year.

This is an old-time method of handling unwanted pregnancies. It would be announced to everyone that the young girl had gone away to a boarding school in a distant state. There were also, to my understanding, certain "shelters" or "convents" for such children, where they accepted youngsters from other states, maintained total secrecy, provided obstetrical care and on-going schooling. In reality, the patient moved from her home for a period of time in order to deliver the baby and put it up for adoption, without anybody in her hometown knowing about it (except what they found out surreptitiously – or learned at a later date).

Is this ethical? Yes, if it does something for the patient (the daughter) and does not violate any societal or legal rules.

However, in today's world of increasing communication and people's widening circle of contacts throughout the country and the world, such a plan would be difficult to carry out. A more acceptable one must be sought.

2. *Arrange for an abortion for her.*

You are immediately faced with a serious heart-rending dilemma. Obviously, whatever way you turn, you will have ethical problems—mainly within yourself. If you make this decision, it means that you are doing a 180° reversal of your previous position, both private and public.

You are being forced to make decisions because of these special circumstances. Changing your position brings reactions (both mild and severe criticism, as well as support) from those who did not accept your past stand and it creates within you much anxiety and agony. Even the anticipation of it will feel devastating.

Choosing this option will depend totally on the source and strength of your convictions. What is ethical for one person in this situation may not be ethical for another. So the decision lies directly with you.

3. *Accept the pregnancy and arrange for an adoption.*

This would seem, on the surface, to be the best option unless objected to by the people involved. You and your family must be prepared for the outside criticism and be willing to accept whatever stigma arises out of this situation -- and it will. It comes down to your choice between Option 1 and Options 2 and 3—there seem to be no other avenues for solution.

Another consideration if you decide to let her deliver is the possibility that the baby could turn out to be mentally defective. This would add further burden to the family if the baby is kept (a lifetime of rearing a defective child) or create difficulty for the family in placing the baby for adoption. This creates an ethical dilemma within an ethical dilemma.

The choice of this option means having a ready explanation for questioners, making special arrangements for schooling for the young girl, seeking arrangements for the adoption (preferably through an agency), arranging for obstetrical and postpartum care and a myriad of smaller problems that may arise

Ethical Considerations

This situation presents an insoluble problem, either from a practical view or an ethical standpoint. You must select what to you is the lesser of two evils.

Obviously, the first dilemma is whether to allow the pregnancy to continue. With this decision come a number of complications and considerations: effects on the patient's health, effects on the patient's psyche, increased possibility of a mentally defective baby, , interference with schooling, embarrassment among her peers and neighbors, embarrassment of the family, financial considerations and a host more. Again, the ethical approach is to try to do the best thing for the patient but none of these return her to her pre-rape status; her life, regardless, is forever changed. Multiple subsequent ethical decisions will have to be made, either way.

The second horn of the dilemma is to allow an abortion. With that, too, come many more ethical dilemmas: the burden for the patient (and the family) of such a procedure, explanation of absences to friends and family, and premature introduction of problems for the young lady. Probably the biggest problem is acceptance of this option, considering all its inherent problems.

One serious consideration is the mental health of the family, whichever option they chose. And especially the patient in view of her age. In every situation of this kind, the smartest medical prescription is to seek advice from multiple sources—psychological, psychiatric, religious, ethical, and experts in all of these fields have experience with such a situations and should contribute their input to the family. After the consultations, the family *and the patient* together should discuss and decide on a course of treatment. Even though she is only 13-years old, from both the emotional and intellectual (and ethical) standpoint, she must be included in the decision-making.

The ethical decision here must take into serious account the family's ethical, moral and religious attitude, family finances, educational considerations and, especially, the physical and mental health of the patient. Once again, ethics attempts to do what is best for the patient, within the bounds of societal and legal restrictions.

Second Opinion

by Stanley E. Grogg, DO, FACOP
Professor of Pediatrics
Oklahoma State University –
Center for Health Sciences

In addition to the need for immediate medical care, including evaluation and treatment of STIs of this adolescent, the long-term consequences of the rape and pregnancy need to be discussed and a plan developed. There are several ethical issues involved with this situation and recommendations will depend on one's moral convictions, peer pressures and perhaps spiritual guidance.

The physician/father has the following options for his daughter. None of them are ideal and without long-term consequence.

1. Send her "away to school" for a year
   a. Keep the baby or
   b. Give the infant up for adoption

There are two options if she were to be sent "away to school" for a year; the family could keep the baby or give the infant up for adoption. Sending the adolescent away for the year to keep a "secret" from her friends and the local "society," could add to the long-term negative effects of the situation. First of all, the family's and friends' support systems would not be easily obtained during the pregnancy. The teenager would most likely feel very lonely and would need to deal with her issues, including medical and psychological, without the support of her family and friends. She would not be able to verbalize her feelings with someone she might trust from her former community.

I would assume that if she were to be away during the pregnancy the infant would be put up for adoption. At some point in time, the situation would most likely "surface" in the physician's and teenager's community and might result in additional psychological and social issues for all concerned. Although a family member might consider assuming the care and financial responsibility of the child, it would not be ideal for the child, mother nor physician/grandfather. I do not feel that sending the pregnant teen off for a year is an appropriate option for this young adult.

2. Arrange for abortion

This is certainly an option if agreed upon by the family and patient. However, if the physician/father has a true conviction against abortions, it would not make sense for him to recommend aborting the fetus. His credibility would be questioned by his colleagues, family members and friends. On the other hand, if the 13-year old, after discussions with perhaps a psychologist or other counselor and family, had a strong desire to have an abortion, then her requests need to be considered. The young pregnant lady would need to understand the potential risks and long-term consequences of an abortion.

3. Accept the pregnancy and arrange for an adoption

This alternative is the most consistent with the physician's previous thoughts and discussions with his peers. There would most likely be long-term consequences for this young lady if she were forced to deliver a live birth and give the child up for adoption. On the other hand, because of her age and maturity level, this could be an acceptable alternative.

I would suggest a 4th option:

4. Accept the pregnancy and keep the infant

The physician/father needs to consider accepting the pregnancy and raising the infant in the family. Alternative schools are available for young mothers to attend and receive proper instruction for the care of children.

Finally, I would like to add two other considerations:

There is a good chance the child will be of normal intelligence even though the biological father is mentally challenged. Ethical issues of who will be financially responsible for the long-term care of the infant will need to be discussed if the mother and family elect to deliver a live birth.

Ethically, the desires of the 13-year-old need to be listened to and understood. Although the physician/father has opposed abortion in the past, his daughter and other family members may not have the same beliefs. Consultation with a psychologist, clergy member and/or other community support systems should be obtained before a final decision is made.

Situation Eleven

A 16-year old girl with acute kidney problems received a transplant kidney from her father. It failed and she was placed on hemodialysis. She tolerated this poorly, vomited constantly, and about 8 months after the dialysis began, she announced, after a lengthy period of illness, that she no longer wanted to be maintained on dialysis. What do you do?

The Options

1. Call her parents.

2. Turn her down.

3. Grant her wish.

4. Initiate conferencing to help her make her final decision.

A Look at the Options

1. Call her parents.

This is one of the few ethical situations with a YES AND NO answer. YES, because the parents must sooner or later (preferably sooner) be aware of her request, so they can help her in this serious and deadly decision. NO, if it's an immediate and impulsive decision without serious thought.

Perhaps the important question here is: How, when and by whom should the parents be told? That answer can only be reached through discussions with the patient, many discussions if needed, and maybe after some consultations. I believe the physician's role and responsibility is to convince the patient to include her parents (and her family) in a total review of her entire situation and give serious consideration for her feelings in the matter. This must be kept in mind throughout all preliminary discussions, but must only be done with her explicit permission.

The parents are already major players in the situation— they decided to get her a kidney transplant, the father donated his kidney, they arranged for the dialysis, they pay for her care, probably provide transportation and coordinate her schooling. Probably in this situation, the patient might be more willing to continue to include them, even though this latest dilemma is such a serious one.

Throughout this review, I have chosen to assume (for clarity) a two-parent family, ignoring the possibility of a single parent family, a divorced family or the existence of no family at all; these would only compound the decision, add confusing ethical considerations and distract us from the impact of the immediate problem.

2. *Turn her down.*

This, too, would be an impulsive reaction, and is not warranted. Maybe later, it could be considered -- maybe not -- but certainly it should not be an immediate action.

Her request is, in effect, a suicide wish—and deserving consideration as a cry for help. This is not the time for clichés, such as "There's always hope", "You are strong. You will get through this", "You're too young to die" and the like. As a cry for help, the response should be something like, "I am here to help you. I hear what you say and I know you are troubled. I also understand what's bothering you. So tell me more about what your feelings are. What are your reasons for wanting to stop therapy? What would be the reasons for continuing it?" That cannot be said and done with one hand on the doorknob to end the visit. Like a patient who develops sudden dyspnea in your office, or faints, immediate care is needed – ethically, medically and legally -- regardless of how busy the doctor is at the moment.

An immediate answer indicates that the physician is making a life and death decision for the young lady, based on the doctor's personal feelings and maybe on incomplete information. We must ask, "Do we have the ethical right to do that, especially impulsively?"

3. Grant her wish.

As an immediate reaction, this is also inappropriate.

At this point, the physician should "take command of the ship" and offer as much help as possible to this troubled girl. It's time to sit down and talk and then move to create a reality situation for her. That probably will call for multiple inputs—from such consultants as pediatrician, nephrologist, ethics specialist, psychiatrist or personal clergy (depending on her wishes). Some people in those fields may have already encountered similar situations and would be of great help in the decision-making—and even have experience in relating and talking to the patient.

4. Initiate conferencing to help her decide.

As alluded to in the other options, this option probably is the only immediate one of value — bringing together those (family and experts) who can help the young, troubled, suffering girl. She apparently sees no way out of her morass, and maybe there is no way out. But that decision must be made exclusively after strong, realistic and intelligent input, information that the young lady most likely does not have or has not considered.

Remember always that this patient can carry out her wish by herself merely by not showing up, by not cooperating or by fighting physically against the dialysis. So if you choose an inappropriate option—on that does not help her—she can go ahead without you. THIS IS A CRY FOR HELP! And obviously she thinks you are the one who might answer it.

Ethical Considerations

This is one situation —maybe more than our other ones — that calls for immediate conferencing, bringing together the patient and her family and involving other experienced experts.

If the medical situation is as deadly as Suzanne feels it is, her desires can be understood. Imagine a 70-year old terminal patient expressing the desire for his life-supports to be discontinued. Understandable. But a 16-year old creates a different scenario. Should she be allowed to ask this? Should we agree with her? Have we the right to force her to continue the "torture" of an unsatisfactory therapy? What are the considerations? Is cure in the prognosis? Probably not? Satisfactory life under treatment? Probably not? Continuation of non-curative (but supportive) treatment that she resents? Probably yes.

Stopping the hemodialysis is like cutting off the life-support of that terminal patient. It means death. It is serious. It is painful to the family (either way). However, it does remove the patient's suffering -- and the hopelessness for the future. What a dilemma!

If the patient is incorrect about her situation (and maybe there really is some hope for a better life), she deserves a great deal of detailed medical information until she fully understands the positive and negative factors in her future.

Ethically, the essential questions (for the physician) are: Is she terminal? Have all avenues been explored? Are we treating for the sake of treating -- or for our own conscience? Or is there some unexplained (or not understood) bright spot in this situation? Is she old enough (and mature enough) for us to give full regard to her wishes?

Are we willing to proceed with her parents' approval -- or without their approval?

All this is difficult in the face of the over-riding definition of ethical care—always do what is best for the *patient.*

Second Opinion

by Samuel K. Snyder, DO, FACOI, FACP, FASN
Chairman, Department of Internal Medicine
Director, Division of Nephrology
College of Osteopathic Medicine
Nova Southeastern University

This unfortunate young woman has reached a point of desperation in the evolution of her disease, plagued by complications, and she desires an end to it all. Compounding these feelings of illness and hopelessness are the complex of emotions she may be experiencing because her failed kidney transplant. This kidney was her father's gift, the kidney he donated, and losing it may be having repercussions on several levels. She wants to discontinue dialysis, to bring an end to her disease and to her life. To examine the ethical dimensions of her problem, we will explore a number of issues, including the following: the nature of death after discontinuation of dialysis; who participates in making this decision; the principles of medical ethics; ethical dimensions of this decision; medical reasons why the patient might tolerate dialysis poorly; medical reasons why the patient might want to discontinue dialysis; non-medical reasons why the patient might want to discontinue dialysis; the effects of the decision on the patient; and the ongoing ethical responsibilities of the caregivers, even if dialysis is discontinued.

When an individual who is completely dialysis-dependent discontinues this life-sustaining modality, death comes within eight or nine days, on average. Most have described it as a painless, even peaceful death. It might occur suddenly, in the middle of the night, because the accumulation of potassium can cause cardiac standstill. Or it might be more gradual in onset, as fluid collects in the lungs, and pulmonary edema causes worsening shortness of breath. The discomfort of this can be treated successfully with drugs such as morphine. Very often, the build-up of waste products and toxins, which had been removed by dialysis, causes gradual lowering of consciousness, and eventually coma. Once this has occurred, death follows inevitably and, it seems, peacefully.

There may clearly be situations where the time seems to have come to discontinue dialysis or other life-sustaining technologies. It is a matter of extreme importance that the patient (if he/she is able) and family or surrogates cooperate in making such a decision, and that they are all fully aware of the consequences and alternatives. A sixteen-year-old should not be left alone with a decision of such magnitude, without input from her family and caregivers, any more than she should be allowed to manage her disease without the guidance of a physician.

Four classical principles of ethical decision making apply. These include beneficence, autonomy, non-maleficence, and the duty of advocacy. The caregiver must honor his obligation to do good and respect life. The caregiver must honor the patient's or surrogate's right to maintain control of the decision-making process. The caregiver must ensure that no harm comes to the patient, as far as possible. And the caregiver must remain an advocate for the patient's well-being.

Making end-of-life decisions is difficult and painful for patients, family members and caregivers. The ethical imperatives that we use to guide us might at times seem to conflict with each other. For instance, is a patient's right to autonomy violated if a caregiver feels that being an advocate means that he/she must always advocate for life? Can the principles of beneficence and non-maleficence be in conflict, when all involved seek to do good for the patient, but doing good involves exposure to side-effects and complications of treatments which the patient tolerates poorly? Hopefully, some of the thoughts that follow will demonstrate that each of these principles can be honored in its turn, as the patient, family and caregivers go through the process of decision making. By the same token, it will be apparent that none of these principles exists in a vacuum, or is totally sacrosanct; but rather, each is conditioned by the other. Thus, even the principle of autonomy is not absolute, and other values and aspects of a particular situation must be taken into account even in consideration of a patient's right to autonomy.

The decision to end dialysis is not to be taken lightly, and it is in the patient's best interest for all to be certain that all alternatives have been explored carefully. In the present case, the caregivers must ask themselves, why does this girl have so many complications with the dialysis procedure? After all, dialysis is well tolerated by hundreds of thousands of people. Can her prescription be modified to make it more tolerable for her? Are her medications part of the problem, and can they be changed or discontinued? If she has been on hemodialysis, perhaps she could benefit from changing modality to peritoneal dialysis, or vice versa. And perhaps a second transplant can be sought, though this takes time, perhaps many months. In other words, can the caregivers reduce the inherent "harm" in the procedure, to give greater benefit to the patient? If they could do so, this might also reduce the patient's wish to die, and still allow her to maintain her autonomy.

When discussing the question, caregivers and family members should feel free to explore with the patient her reasons for wanting to stop dialysis. Often in the case of patients on dialysis this is readily apparent. But it is a question that deserves review, because it might save a life whose end is premature. Does our patient want to stop dialysis just because she feels sick, as discussed above? Perhaps if the caregivers could find medical ways to alleviate the symptoms, the patient might change her mind. Often chronically ill patients are depressed, and that can strongly color their decision making. The patient and caregivers should explore whether a trial of antidepressant medication and counseling should be undertaken before irrevocable decisions are made.

Are there emotional components to her decision that, while not medical per se, have impacted on her condition? In this case, what might be going through the mind of a sixteen-year-old girl who knows that her father has given her a precious gift, his own kidney, and that it has failed? Might she have feelings of failure herself? Perhaps she sees her own death as the way out of feelings of guilt for having lost her father's kidney. Patients seek meaning in their illness. Family and caregivers can help guide them in finding the most appropriate meaning. In this case, any sense of guilt for the transplant's failure is a meaning that should be denied and refuted. Certainly, she must be made aware that these feelings are far from the truth of her medical situation, and really have no relevance to her father's true feelings for her. She should not feel responsible in any sense for her own illness; every effort should be made to dissuade her from taking action on the basis of these feelings.

Are outside emotional factors at play? The teen years are turbulent, even for healthy kids. Serious illness can affect an adolescent's relationships with peers. During those years, the most emotionally vulnerable of our children are at risk for bad decisions because of emotional confusion; and for the most vulnerable of them, these decisions can go as far as suicide. It is vitally important that any issues in this area be explored, and that the patient be counseled about them. It is inappropriate to make a life or death choice about discontinuation of dialysis on the basis of these kinds of problems, which—although they are very real to the patient—are extraneous to the medical decision-making at hand.

Even though the patient might decide to end her life by discontinuing dialysis, this decision itself changes the character of her illness. It is like receiving news of having a terminal disease all over again. Thus, it is important for family and caregivers to anticipate that the patient might go through the stages described by Elisabeth Kubler-Ross in coming to grips with her own decision. These include denial, anger, depression, bargaining and acceptance. The family and caregiver should try to help the patient move through these stages before irrevocable action is taken, so that the patient can achieve the greatest level of peace that is possible.

It is the obligation of the caregivers to guide the patient and family through the process, with all the considerations discussed above. There are probably others as well, for every situation of life and death has its own features unique to the individual involved. Even with the ongoing involvement of family, the patient's autonomy can be respected. By the same token, the family must be included in this process, for their sake and the sake of the patient.

If the patient does finally decide to stop dialysis, knowing she will die soon, the caregivers' ethical responsibilities don't end. Certainly this is a terrible decision. There are guidelines that can help us through terrible medical decisions, which the caregivers must carry out. When a person is dying, especially if he or she is in pain, any intervention that prolongs dying may be rejected or discontinued. When there is no reasonable hope of improvement, treatment that prolongs or causes pain may be rejected or discontinued. Pain must be treated as aggressively as possible. Impediments to dying should be removed. And finally, there are situations in which acceptance of death is in the best interest of the patient.

This approach ensures that the patient has the last word. And yet it also offers the patient every opportunity to choose to continue in life. Ultimately, every human being needs a sense of purpose in order to choose life over death. If our patient could glean no other purpose for continuing her treatment after going through this process than ongoing pain and suffering—living in order to dialyze, rather than dialyzing in order to live—then, it might be the best thing for her family and caregivers to support her in her decision, and ease her passage to death. On the other hand, this process can give the patient an opportunity to find new purpose, and to continue life. Either way, she deserves the complete support of her family and caregivers.

Situation Twelve

Suzanne, age 16, comes to your office and requests that you place her on contraceptive medication, as she is sexually active. You explain that you feel that you cannot do this. She then says that, since she knows no one else to turn to, she will sue you for wrongful pregnancy, if she ever becomes pregnant.

The Options

1. Call her parents.

2. Advise her to stop having sex.

3. Prescribe the contraceptives and tell her not to return.

4. Refer her to Planned Parenthood or a similar service.

5. Prescribe contraceptive as she requested.

A Look at the Options

1. Call her parents.

We have already exhausted in several previous situations all the reasons that this is not really a viable option. Confidentiality, privacy, confidence – all the factors given before apply as strongly in this case. Plus, it will serve no purpose and solve no problems, but only create havoc. So rule this out.

2. Advise her to stop having sex.

This is impossible on the face of it. Telling a 16-year old to stop having sex just because you say so (even if you give reasons) is like telling someone not to think of the word "hippopotamus" for the next five minutes. It just won't work, and I doubt that any sophisticated questioner would ever suggest this.

3. Prescribe the contraceptives and tell her not to return.

Prescribing under these circumstances may solve your problem for the moment, and maybe even convince the young lady that you are helping her. Without sufficient knowledge, she might believe that she will just renew the medication as needed, or she may have some other simplistic rationale for accepting this.

However, for you the implications are multiple. First, dismissing her without her having another physician is obvious abandonment—and no doctor wants that charge. Second, the abandonment leaves the patient with no recourse in case of renewal, complications, further education or any unforeseen circumstances.

Besides the words you say, your attitude and deportment must exude professionalism. You must explain carefully to her why you will not be continuing as her doctor. Your "dismissal" should not be abrupt or hostile. This must follow all ethical precepts.

4. *Refer her to Planned Parenthood or a similar service.*

Ethically and logically, this is a suitable and fair alternative if you do not wish to continue. But it must be done in a tone of helping this young lady. She should understand the work and attitude of the clinic, and be aware of your desire to help her. You need to explain carefully why you are referring her, what the role and status of Planned Parenthood is, and what services and help they will provide.

As a supportive service to your patient and as a demonstration to her of your willingness to help, you might consider calling Planned Parenthood yourself to explain the circumstances and set up an appointment for her. After all, at 16, she may not have the sophistication, or knowledge or mind-set to do this herself — and you certainly would not want her to leave your office without a definite follow-up.

5. Prescribe contraceptives, as she requested.

This is a good solution, provided it is part of a complete therapeutic visit. In spite of her age (or maybe because of it), the physician must do a complete initial "contraceptive" visit: whatever medical history is needed, whatever physical examination is indicated (including gynecological), and whatever guidance or psychological support is needed, as well as instructions in the use of the contraceptive medication, how and when to use refills and possible complications. For any of these that are not in your realm of practice, be sure to get consultation or make a referral. You should arrange for a follow-up visit as you usually do and be sure she understands what changes should bring her back to your office.

It would be wise and ethically important to discuss with her the importance of involving her parents and the benefits of their knowing—including how to tell them. Again, involving yourself would be a greatly supportive measure. If need be, your calling her parents to set up an appointment to discuss their daughter's medical problem would be a good introduction to your sitting down in a group discussion with the patient and her parents, so you can introduce the topic. This also enables you to control the discussion and prevent hostile parent-child disputes. This move would greatly strengthen (with your input and help) the parent-child relationship and, at the same time, enhance the doctor-patient relationship.

This solution seems to offer the best and most ethical possibility for guiding this young lady into a workable option for her problem.

Ethical Considerations

There are three special considerations in this situation, and all three have impact on the ethical aspects:

Influence of the Internet. Gone are the days when we would assume that a 16-year old was totally unsophisticated in sex and contraception.

With all our modern education and growth in communication, many of our children probably come to us with greater knowledge (and misconceptions) of sex than generations ago. While the amount of knowledge is variable among children, for the most part they do have a reasonable understanding of sex.

Today's communication advances, specifically the Internet, can provide as much information, and in depth, about contraceptives as the young people want to know. (Google, for example has 30 million citations for contraception, and Yahoo has over 12 million). And we must assume, therefore, that many of the young people will come to us with substantially more factual knowledge than a generation ago. And especially a sexually-active 16-year old who had to decide consciously to visit you with her request. That means you must use a different approach, and have a high ethical regard, and respect, for the patients and their knowledge.

Medical complications. To avoid confusing the discussions, consideration of medical complications have not been covered. Suffice it to say that all of us have a realization that common adolescent problems, such as depression, thoughts of suicide, suicide itself and the many implications of substance abuse must always be kept in mind. These medical complications multiply the ethical considerations for the doctor.

The threat of "wrongful pregnancy" lawsuit. While the threat of lawsuit from the patient may be serious or kidding, physicians must always keep it in the back of their minds. "Wrongful pregnancy" is an accepted and tried action at law—used in many instances such as misinformation about pregnancy or the fetus, botched abortion or abdominal surgery, unsatisfactory tubal ligation, or some negligence leading eventually to pregnancy. It has been roughly defined as negligence leading to the birth of a healthy baby, but unwanted and unplanned.

There are no reported cases, as far as I can tell, of "wrongful pregnancy" arising from a physician's failure to prescribe contraceptives on request. Since it has been said, maybe semi-facetiously, that anyone can sue anybody for any reason, it is logical to assume that some day someone will try this route for a lawsuit—and physicians should be aware of the possibility. (Yahoo has over 600,000 citations for "wrongful pregnancy.") Again, this potential legal challenge adds to the ethical considerations.

Second Opinion

by Sandy D. Melnick, MD
Attending Psychiatrist
Director of Outpatient Psychotherapy
Chester-Crozer Medical Center

I must ask: Why did the doctor refuse? Is the patient too young? Too immature? Did the doctor not know how to comfortably handle whether or how to involve her parents?

I would also want to ask questions about the doctor. At what age did the doctor first have sex and with whom? What was the age of his/her partner? Why did he/she do it then? Was birth control used? Disease prevention? How might all these things affect his/her point of view? Is he/she asking the patient to be different than the doctor was? Why? Or the same? Why?

In general, doctors need to guard against being too self-righteous as if they know best for everyone about everything, and as if they have the right to impose their particular ideas on others. What makes their ideas more "right" or "wise" than the next person? Have their own lives been so perfect in the decisions that were made? Is what was right for them therefore right for everyone?

The only way to be sure that you won't be sued is to give up clinical practice. So, let's leave out the legal issues and focus on the ethics involved.

We also want to know the attitude of her and her parents about this situation? With adolescent patients, it is wise to have a general discussion with them ahead of time. Establish, I think, that you would like your door always to be open in a confidential way and that there can be confidential contacts between you and the adolescent. Establish that you may provide information or treatment without telling the parents, if that's what's necessary to create the availability of another stable and responsible adult in her life. If she needs to reach out to you, there's probably a good reason. Also establish that certain types of information or situations will have to be communicated to the parents, with an understanding at the outset what these might be. Ideally, come up with guidelines, together with the patient and her parents, that all parties find comfortable or at least acceptable.

Coming back to the present situation, this patient wouldn't be coming to you unless she is already sexually active or has already made up her mind to start having sex. Realistically, even if you are opposed to it, you at this point have no ability to control her decision. Acting as if you have power that you don't have helps no one. Remember, "First, do no harm." Shutting doors accomplishes nothing. Instead, use the opportunity to open doors.

By being receptive to her request, you have an opportunity for on-going discussion and counseling. Let her know you will honor her request, but couple this with a need to talk some more. Make open-ended inquiries. Why does this come up now? Is she already having sex? Who is the intended (or already) partner? Why him? What is the nature of the relationship? Is this a mutual decision that she (and he) is comfortable with? Or is she (or he) getting pressured? What does she know about sex, pregnancy, birth control, STDs, etc.? Take the opportunity to teach her and to draw out and discuss her feelings.

See what role her parents could take and if she'd allow it. If it's okay with her, meet with them all together and help them talk.

Find excuses for follow-up appointments. Meet again to provide further education. Have a "check-up" after the first sexual encounter, to continue general discussion as well as to address any feelings or problems that may have arisen. Follow up just to see how things are going so far. If you prescribe an oral contraceptive, this will delay any sex (if she follows instructions) for a month, until a full cycle goes by. In the interim, meet more, assess side effects (and talk!).

If you are uncomfortable or unskilled with this sort of counseling, I would suggest getting some "supervision" for yourself, from a psychiatrist or other mental health professional. The patient came to YOU, so she trusts and respects you. Don't be too quick to refer her away, possibly implying to her that you are rejecting her and seeing her as mentally ill. Over time, an opportunity for a referral may arise comfortably. If you do make a referral, especially if it is early on, I would emphasize that this must be an expert (make sure he/she actually is) on educating about sex and helping people make decisions about the role of sex in their lives. (By the way, statistically, those people who are best educated about sex tend to be less promiscuous and tend to make more conservative decisions about sexual behavior.)

Epilogue

So much is controversial and confusing about ethical problems. Interpretation of what is and what is not ethical depends on our backgrounds, our experiences, our training, and yes, our prejudices, bad or good. Unfortunately, some interpretations of ethics are based on personal whim, or greed, or the "what's in it for me" syndrome.

I thought long about this in reviewing the problem cases I've included in this book. Rarely the poet, I found that form of expression best to explain concisely what all of us should think about whenever we encounter an ethical situation or think that some situation has ethical aspects.

I hope it makes you think!

I Wonder

<ins>I Wonder</ins>

I wonder why my ethics are right and your ethics are wrong.

<ins>I Wonder</ins>

I wonder: if ethics are standards, and standards are absolutes, and absolutes are rules, and rules are unbending. I wonder if that's ethical.

<ins>I Wonder</ins>

I wonder if ethics is really tunnel-visioned
I wonder if <ins>only</ins> society is important, or <ins>only</ins> the individual is important, or <ins>only</ins> the family- is important.
I wonder if that's ethics.

<ins>I Wonder</ins>

I wonder if I had been born in a different country, would my ethics be different.
I wonder if I had been born in 1890 or in 2090, would my ethics be different.
I wonder how I -- or you --can be sure.

<ins>I Wonder</ins>

I wonder as a physician, faced with a problem that is family-sundering or heart-rending or life-threatening, can

anyone climb into my brain--or into my responsibility--
and tell me what to do.

I wonder, when I face that problem, do I have the
unfettered right to solve it my own way.

I Wonder

I wonder why we call it ethics -- ethics should solve
problems.

I wonder whether we should call it dilemma, cause
that's the burden it places on us.

I Wonder, I Wonder, I Wonder